D0426924

Winning in the Women's Health Care Marketplace

Genie James

Winning in the Women's Health Care Marketplace

A Comprehensive Plan for Health Care Strategists

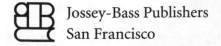

Jossey-Bass Publishers
San Francisco

Jossey-Bass books and products are available through most bookstores. To contact Jossey-Bass directly, call (888) 378–2537, fax to (800) 605–2665, or visit our website at www.josseybass.com.

Substantial discounts on bulk quantities of Jossey-Bass books are available to corporations, professional associations, and other organizations. For details and discount information, contact the special sales department at Jossey-Bass.

 Manufactured in the United States of America on Lyons Falls Turin Book. This paper is acid-free and 100 percent totally chlorine-free.

Library of Congress Cataloging-in-Publication Data

James, Genie.
    Winning in the women's health care marketplace: a comprehensive plan for health care strategists/Genie James.
        p. cm.
    Includes bibliographical references and index.
    ISBN 0-7879-4444-0 (alk. paper)
    1. Women's health services—Economic aspects. 2. Women's health services—Social aspects. 3. Women—Health and hygiene. I. Title.
    RA564.85.J35   1999
    338.4'3362198—dc21   99-38980
                                                                                                            CIP

FIRST EDITION
HB Printing   10 9 8 7 6 5 4 3 2 1

⸻ Contents

*To my sister, Sheila Hardeman, because I love you
and want us both to be healthy, live a very long time,
share all the good things life offers along the way,
and laugh a whole lot more!*

*To my sisters in spirit, Gayle Alexander,
Nan Allison, Pam Baggett, Diane Bush, Margaret Deal,
Kerry Eason, Cynthia Enger, Sue Fort-White,
Pat Glaser-Shea, Stacy Graham, Robin Growden,
Leah Hall, Nancy McMorrow, Corrine Matthews,
Karen Miller, Roxie Phillips, Mary Schmidt,
Jan Hulme Shepard, Connie Tatgenhorst,
Anne Vincent, Suzie Waters-Benjamin,
Denise Weiss, and Vicki Yenzer,
because you have all helped me learn to love myself.*

*To my niece, Shelley Hardeman, because you teach about living
and I celebrate the exquisite woman you are becoming.*

~~~ Preface

The issue of women's health is not new. Why, then, is it now important for health care business executives to reexamine it? The reasons are clear. Women's health combines the three most important challenges facing today's health care leaders:

- The need to capture more covered lives and increase market share
- The need to protect revenue streams via referrals and new retail strategies
- The need to insert social consciousness into an aggressive profit-driven strategy for health services delivery

Every senior-level executive within a health system has a very real dictate to meet these challenges.

Once I began to research women's health as more than gender-specific medicine, I was excited to realize that women are a market force that has the power and motivation to reshape the health care delivery system. I want the information in this book to help professionals and decision makers realize the importance of women as consumers of health care.

When I first decided to write this book, I was executive vice president of managed care and marketing for an OB/GYN physician practice management firm. I made no claims to be an expert on women's health. What I was—and am—is a business strategist with a skill set that enables me to do the following:

- Identify trends and market forces
- Evaluate the impact of these on the critical business objectives of market share and revenue

- Respond with entrepreneurial and intrapreneurial strategies to maximize performance within a changing reality
- Develop and oversee management plans for action and implementation

Winning in the Women's Health Care Marketplace extends well beyond my research and skills. It also draws on the voices and experience of many leaders in the burgeoning field of women's health. The experts cited here—more than a dozen of them, all with extensive knowledge about women's health care issues and opportunities—make the book come alive in a way I hope helps redefine women's health.

This book is not theoretical. Hard data and statistics validate recommended strategies. Part One educates the reader about trends, market dynamics, and political variables that draw women's health to the forefront. Chapters One and Two give an overview of the women's health marketplace and a sense of the important role of women through the years. Chapters Three and Four explain women's clout as consumers and players in the health care market. Chapter Five discusses adapting product lines and information technology for women consumers today and tomorrow.

In Part Two, the importance of women's health is integrated with the most pressing issues facing health care leaders today. Chapter Six discusses success factors for providers of women's health services, and Chapter Seven, the women's health market and the private sector. Integrated systems of care for women's health are covered in Chapter Eight, followed by the social reconnaissance approach in Chapter Nine. The underserved in health care are discussed in Chapter Ten, and Chapter Eleven covers getting the most from every marketing dollar.

If you think that money is more important to the system than patient care, see Part Three. It highlights the caregiver and emphasizes an aggressive approach to preventive medicine and case management. The joint-equity model of physician integration and the nurse practitioner model are covered in Chapters Twelve and Thirteen. The burgeoning consumer demand for a whole-person approach to medical treatment is addressed in Chapters Fourteen through Sixteen. Chapter Seventeen focuses on Medicare and the women's health market. Chapter Eighteen stresses the advent and benefits of a more relationship-centered approach to patient care.

Those of us in the health care industry are witnessing a period of deep-seated change that can be very positive for patient and provider alike. The approaches and strategies in this book give you some innovative ideas and help you recognize that women's health is integral to your key business objectives—now and for the future.

Nashville, Tennessee   GENIE JAMES
October 1999

~~~ Acknowledgments

The substance of this book has been derived from the knowledge of a small team of experts. I am grateful to them all for their willingness to share their knowledge and for their kindness in nudging me forward. Many thanks to the following:

The National Association for Women's Health (NAWH); Cliff Adlerz, COO, SYMBION Healthcare; Nan Allison, Allison & Beck Nutrition Consulting; David Balloff, Aviation Subcommittee, U.S. House of Representatives; William G. Bates, M.D.; Marianne Bouldin, a principal of Taylor Hill Communications; Maxine Brinkman, director of women's services, North Iowa Mercy Health Network; Cheryl Carlson, former CEO of Echelon Health; Donna Cheek, executive director of YWCA Nashville; Yonnie Chesley, president of Gordian Health Solutions, Inc.; Marjean Coddon, vice president of the Learning Institute, Quorum Health Resources, LLC; Colleen Conway-Welch, Vanderbilt University School of Nursing; Sue Fort-White, resource development specialist of Oasis Center, Inc.; Marlene von Friederichs–Fitzwater, director of the Health Communication Research Institute, Inc.; Pat Glaser-Shea, former COO of Echelon Health, Inc.; Stacey Graham, marketing and communications consultant; Bill Hamburg, president and CEO of Medisphere Health Partners, Inc.; Michael Heard, vice president of integration services, Quorum Health Resources, LLC; Steve Hines, M.D.; and Della M. Hughes, executive director of the National Network for Youth.

Also, Wanda Jones, Ph.D., deputy assistant secretary for health, U.S. Department of Health and Human Services; Susan Kuner, Ed.D., Virtual School/University Relations, Vanderbilt University; Betty Larsen, M.S.W., The Yoga Room; Gregg O. Lehman, president and CEO of the National Business Coalition on Health; Cathy Strachan Lindenburg, R.N., Ph.D., at the University of Washington School of Nursing; R. Clayton McWhorter, chairman of Clayton Associates, LLC; Michele M. Molden, executive vice president of product line management and strategic planning, Olympic Health Management Systems; Cyndy Nayer, principal at River City Partnership on Health, Inc.; Amy Niles, executive director of the National Women's Health Resource Center; Kathleen Pittman, D.S.N., R.N.C., P.N.P., and assistant professor of child and adolescent health at Georgia State University School of Nursing; and Joanne F. Pulles, executive director of Nashville Healthcare Partnership, Partners for a Healthy Nashville.

Also, Elizabeth "Buffy" Reicht, director of community policy for the Arizona governor's office; Sally Rynne, president of Rynne Marketing Group; Marie Shaw, director of women's health services at Lehigh Valley Hospital; Dave Sluyter, M.D. and vice president of education at the Fetzer Institute; Roxanne Spitzer, professor and associate dean at the Vanderbilt University School of Nursing; Ronnie Steine, CEO of Oasis Center, Inc.; Cheryl Stone, senior vice president of Rynne Marketing Group; Marcia Twitty, director of marketing and public relations for Baptist Health System, Inc., in Birmingham, Alabama; Debbie Wells, policy adviser on health for the Arizona governor's office; Tracey Wimberly, senior vice president of missions, Baptist Health System, in Nashville, Tennessee; and Mary Wooley, president of Research! America.

Special thanks to the chapter contributors, whose efforts make the book reach as far as it does: Ann Boeke, M.S., C.H.E., and former director of Women's Ambulatory Initiatives at Mercy Health System; Jim Burdine, principal at Felix, Burdine & Associates; Michael Felix, principal at Felix, Burdine & Associates; Stacy Graham, marketing and communications consultant; Kathleen Hanold, R.N., M.S., and vice president of women and infant services in the BJC Health System; Cathy Hoot, writer, consultant, and principal of Cathy Hoot & Associates; John Kaszuba, manager of the Learning Institute, Quorum Health Resources, LLC; Rita Menitoff, founder and president of Women's Health Management Solutions, LLC; Holly Owens, RFP team manager for TCS Management Group; Jeffrey Persson, senior manager of integration services for the Horne CPA Group; Laura Reed, freelance writer and consultant; Jaynelle Stichler, D.N.S. and principal of the Stichler Group, Inc.; and Kim Weiss, consultant with BDC Advisors, LLC, and former executive director of the NAWH.

Having gathered material from experts in health care, I then called on publishing experts to turn this wealth of information into a book. Numerous reviewers and editors offered guidance along the way. Two freelance developmental editors, Audrey Kaufman and Jan Hunter, recommended changes to the organization and structure, rewrote sections, pushed for more information, and generally improved the book. Andy Pasternack, senior editor at Jossey-Bass, held and nurtured the idea for this book through many changes; he was ably assisted by Katie Crouch, editorial assistant. Gigi Mark and Susan Geraghty, production editors, saw the manuscript through the production process. Danielle Neary, assistant marketing manager, and Margaret Sebold, director of marketing, then brought the finished book to shelves and screens for purchase. Finally, this book could not have moved from concept to printed work without the assistance of Judy McCaskill, who worked many long hours to take my notes and get them into readable, usable form. To all the people who played a key role in the development of this book, I offer my heartfelt thanks.

G.J.

⟿ The Author

Genie James, M.M.Sc., is a consultant and author whose energies are focused on strategic business development and the launch of new programs and products. For the past decade, James has operated primarily in the health care sector, working with health systems, physician groups, and investor communities to move concepts from inception to implementation. Anticipating that shifting patterns of health care reimbursement might create opportunities for new models of care, James has devoted herself to examining emerging trends in health management, holistic medicine, e-commerce, and women's health services. Her innovative thought and approach are evident in her first book, *Making Managed Care Work* (Irwin, 1997), and this book, her second.

Winning in the Women's Health Care Marketplace

The Health Care Gatekeepers

Women Hold the Keys

Part One explores in depth the women's health marketplace and women's role in creating, changing, and driving the field. In Chapter One, John Kaszuba describes the power women hold as gatekeepers to health care and the importance of providing for women's health care throughout life.

The history of the women's health movement, from its roots in early feminism to the present, is discussed in Chapter Two. People today live longer, and women are an increasing majority of that older population. Health care decision makers face many questions today; Chapter Three looks at how public policy, legislative action, and women's health issues interrelate. Women's strength as consumers and their influence on public policy and how health dollars are spent is covered in Chapter Four. Chapter Five takes this information into the future: how best to adapt products and information technology for the consumers of today and tomorrow.

CHAPTER ONE

Understanding the Women's Health Marketplace

John Kaszuba

> *John Kaszuba is manager of the Learning Institute for*
> *Quorum Health Resources, LLC, based in Brentwood,*
> *Tennessee. He is widely recognized as a researcher tracking*
> *market trends and identifying successful health care*
> *entrepreneurial ventures.*

he next time you are at the airport, shopping, or just driving around, look at the people around you. You may observe that there are many more active people over sixty now than when you were growing up. It's true: in industrialized nations people live longer than ever before. Since the beginning of the twentieth century, average life expectancy has increased by more than twenty-five years.

Also, people aged sixty-five live five years longer on average than they did a few years ago, and they don't stand still. Consider, for example, John Glenn, who in 1962 became the first American astronaut to orbit the earth. He returned to space in November 1998 at age seventy-seven as a space shuttle mission specialist.

This increase in life span, compounded with population increases over the past century, means that old people are a larger proportion of the population today. In many industrialized nations, the most rapidly growing age group is that aged eighty and above, and in some countries those over one hundred.[1] This is not to imply that hundred-year-olds will soon dominate the population, but people over eighty are increasing very rapidly. We Americans are living longer. So might our children, and if so they will push the average life expectancy even higher.

People today seem to live longer and to lead healthier lives. But the population of elderly people is still relatively small. What impact, then, does this have on the health marketplace in general and on women's health in particular?

In the United States, as in most industrialized nations, women live about seven years longer than men.[2] As women grow older, they make up an increasingly large portion of the population. In 1990, for example, there were three elderly women for every two elderly men.[3] Census Bureau data for 1992 show that nearly half of the women who reach age sixty-five live to age eighty-five, whereas less than a third of men aged sixty-five do so.[4]

But living longer doesn't necessarily mean that women are healthier when old. Reports from Japan, the United States, and Europe show that even though people are living healthier longer, women spend about twice as many years disabled before death as their male counterparts. That is bad news for women, and also indicates a very real consumer need. Need equals demand, and the health care industry is in business to meet it.

The Bureau of Labor projects that the largest age groups in 2005 will be those aged forty-five to sixty-four (36 percent of the population), fourteen to twenty-four (14 percent), and sixty-five and older (8 percent.) Interestingly, by 2005 the number of people aged twenty-five to forty-four are expected to decrease by 6 percent.

Health care providers would be wise to focus on the heavy demands they face now, most of which will only increase in the future because of these changing demographics. People live longer now, and health care providers must better understand the population they will serve in the coming years if they are to provide the best service. They must also pay attention to advances in medicine and health—which are among the reasons people now live so long.

Also, providers must understand another variable in the supply-and-demand equation: profit management. The shrinking reimbursement dollar means that utilization is not always a good thing. The questions become: How can we deliver the best service, at the best price, at the best time? How can we facilitate appropriate and cost-effective utilization of health services?

WOMEN: AN ECONOMIC FORCE

Women make up a significant portion of the workforce. Those in the health care industry must recognize that women comprise the vast majority of employees, from nurses and clerical personnel to senior executives.

In 1970, 35 percent of women worked part-time and 16 percent full-time. Now 22 percent work part-time and 47 percent full-time. In 1970, 51 percent of working women were mothers. Today they make up 69 percent. Fifty-three percent of working women who get pregnant today are back at work before their baby's first birthday.[5] Working women and mothers are here to stay, in part because in today's economy it commonly takes two earners in a family to achieve a middle-class lifestyle.

Women today are better educated than in previous generations and play a more significant role in the economy. Even by 1990, women were earning 47 percent of all business degrees, 71 percent of psychology degrees, 84 percent of health degrees, and 51 percent of life sciences degrees.[6]

Better education means better pay. A fifth of working women today earn $50,000 a year or more.[7] In addition to holding more and better-paying jobs and being better educated, women are making a monumental impact on the American enterprise system. Unfulfilled or disillusioned with the corporate world, more and more women are choosing to become the employer rather than the employee. According to the National Foundation for Women Business Owners, women now own eight million businesses, about a third of all total American enterprise.[8]

Managed care has forced health care payors and providers to acknowledge that women are a significant market force. As employees, they often drive decisions about benefit plans and provider selection. As employers, they often choose the health plan for their organization.

A major premise of many managed health care plans is that the gatekeepers to health care are the primary care physicians. But health care is a highly competitive, service-based industry that offers many choices. Thus customers are the true gatekeepers. But which customers? Consider the following statistics:

- Women visit doctors and hospital outpatient departments 5.6 times per year versus 2.3 times for men.[9]

- Women are the major consumers of health care in the United States, accounting for 59 percent of prescription drug purchases, 61 percent of doctors' visits, and 66 percent of procedures in hospitals each year.[10]

- Women account for 65 percent of the nation's annual medical bills.[11]

- Women experience a 20 to 30 percent higher incidence of acute illness than men.[12]

- Of the twenty most common surgeries, eleven are done solely on women.[13]

- Almost all autoimmune diseases are more common in women, by a 9-to-1 ratio.[14]

- Two-thirds of all hospital procedures are performed on women, as are seven of the ten most frequently performed surgeries in the United States. For example, more than six hundred thousand hysterectomies are performed each year.[15]

Women are the true gatekeepers to health care. They make 70 to 90 percent of all health care decisions.[16] They make 90 percent of all calls to physician referral and health information services, and are twice as likely to change health care providers if they are dissatisfied with service.[17] Educated working women have substantially increased their buying power and clout, and directly influence how and where much of the American health care dollar is spent. Women typically oversee the health care of their family, both immediate and extended. They tend to be better informed about health than men. Typically, women influence the use of health care services by being the initiators of wellness, prevention, and early intervention for immediate families; referral sources for coworkers, friends, and family; and decision makers for extended families.

Catching health problems at an early stage was considered very important for 90 percent of women surveyed in a Kaiser Family Foundation study.[18] When asked about their single most important attribute in a health plan, 42.5 percent named high-quality care; 93.6 percent think it is "very important" for a health plan to provide high-quality care (97.7 percent of women agree that it is "important"). Nineteen percent of women ranked having a wide range of doctors as the most important selection criteria; 17 percent selected low cost. It seems that the average woman is concerned more with quality and not so much with the number of physicians a plan offers or its cost (although, to be sure, these factors are still important). This shouldn't be a surprise; it's basic consumer behavior. Therefore, to be successful, a health plan or hospital doesn't necessarily need to offer an abundance of physicians, but to lock in those who are the most-asked-for or are perceived to be the best.

These facts alone are enough to proclaim women as health care's main customers. That is further validated considering that women also use health services more than men and will continue to do so in increasing numbers over the next two decades. Being attuned to women's needs both for themselves and for others then becomes key to thriving in the health marketplace.

ADAPTING TO TODAY'S MARKET

How can your health care organization thrive today and tomorrow? Simple: listen, hear, and fulfill. Is your organization really in tune with its customer base? Health care is a service industry and, like any business in a service industry, providers need to determine their target customer segment, what services are needed and valued by that segment, and how and where the customers prefer services to be delivered. If you can't do it, the customers will find someone who can.

Women are a prime example. Today they are vocal about their needs, adopt self-care regimens, turn increasingly toward pharmacists and other sources as partners in preventive health management, exercise more and eat better, and choose therapies in addition to those mainstream medical providers offer. Women are taking charge of their lives, asking more questions, demanding more answers. Doctors, nurses, hospitals, and pharmacists should respect that; women will go elsewhere if they don't. How the health care industry delivered services in the past doesn't count; women clearly demonstrate that they will give their business to providers who can align service delivery with the needs of a whole person, family, or community.

Thus providers must rethink tradition, especially when considering the location and atmosphere where they offer services. Consider the phenomenon of women turning to their OB/GYN for general checkups, screenings, immunizations, and counseling: in other words, for primary care in addition to traditional gynecological and obstetrical services. A 1993 poll[19] found that 54 percent of women who routinely go to OB/GYNs consider them their primary care provider. Probably they feel that OB/GYNs spend more time with them and do a thorough physical exam, discuss lifestyle and preventive health issues, and really understand not only their physical state but also what is happening in their lives. Women may feel that their OB/GYN is more in tune with their health issues than primary care physicians they have seen in the past.

Another recent phenomenon challenging the traditional delivery setting is the retail opportunities associated with women's health care. Retail boutiques that cater to women with various health care needs—from cancer, incontinence, and breast feeding to massage therapy, aromatherapy, and natural treatment clinics—are springing up nationwide and offer a variety of customized services, supplies, and professional support. Also, diagnostic services are popping up in malls. Nordstrom, for example, understanding its customers' health care needs and demand for convenient services, is providing mammography and bone density screenings in its stores.[20] Some popular women's health care programs currently offered in the marketplace include stand-alone women's health centers; multispecialty centers such as sports-fitness and medical "second-opinion" programs; diagnostic centers with services that include mammography, bone density testing, and general radiology; and holistic care centers offering an array of services to treat the mind, body, and spirit.

Not new, but newly discussed, are the differences in delivery of health care to various sectors of the population. Many social issues influence this; one is how minority women are treated. A recent Boston University study exploring minority gender bias by providers reported that at every income level, African-American women over age sixty-four are half as likely as whites to have a mammogram ordered for them by a physician, even when seeing a primary care physician equally as often. The report also stated that mammography rates are even lower for Native American women. For African-American and Native American women, the bottom line is that, although the disease is much less common among them than in whites, they have a 30 percent higher risk of dying of breast cancer.[21] Beth Israel Hospital in Boston conducted a study that concluded that doctors ordered 1.5 times as much surgery and other high-tech treatment for whites as for equally ill African-Americans.[22] According to Colin McCord, associate director of surgery at Harlem Hospital in New York City, "Statistics show that an African-American woman born in Harlem today has less chance of surviving to age 65 than a woman from

Bangladesh, one of the poorest nations on earth."[23] How can this be if our country is the most medically advanced in the world? The answer to that question is not found in the "how" but rather the "why."

To win in the women's health care marketplace, providers must listen to what women of all ages and races want and expect. Traditional OB/GYN services are not enough. Although women may rely on OB/GYNs for a range of services, more and more opt to start families later in life. So providers should consider membership programs, tiered programs, and consumer-specific campaigns that target customers' actual purchasing behavior. And they need to develop programs and services that target women's needs during their stages of life—from early adulthood to middle age to seniority. Such strategies are most likely the ones that will allow providers to keep women as customers for as long as possible. And that is the bottom line: best care for women at all stages of life equals best revenue for health care providers.

LIFE SEGMENTS AND HEALTH CONCERNS

A life segment is an age range within a woman's life that lends itself to categorization of attitudes, concerns, and health risks common to a majority of women within it (see Exhibit 1.1). Simply put, their attitudes and concerns tend to coincide with their life segment, and understanding each stage is important to understanding women as customers. Life span segmentation is a topic of interest today for both medical professionals and consumers.

Medical professionals must race to keep up with the educated consumer. Women readily learn health information through the media. In 1999, *Newsweek, Time, Delicious,* and the *New York Times* were among the host of periodicals running special issues specifically addressing women's health concerns. The following sections briefly present the defining age segments in a woman's life, and the accompanying Exhibits (1.2–1.6), contributed by Bill Bates, provide further detail on the life span segmentation of women's health from a physician's perspective.

The Twenties

Women in their late teens and twenties often think they can have it all and do it all because any consequences lie in the future. They feel invincible, and that keeps many from bothering to learn about preventative

- *Menopause.* By 2000, more than fifty million American women will be at or beyond the age of menopause (forty-eight to fifty-two years). Only about 10 to 20 percent are on continuing hormone replacement therapy. Baby boomers are reaching menopause at a rate of more than two thousand per day.[49] In the United States, more than thirty million women have passed menopause.[50]
- *Depression.* Depression affects 20 percent of the female population in the developed world. In America, 12 percent of women (versus 6 percent of men) have suffered from clinically significant depression at some point.[51] First onset of depression often occurs during a women's most productive years, ages eighteen to forty-four. Primary care doctors still fail to diagnose as many as 50 percent of patients experiencing major depression.[52]
- *Cardiovascular disease.* One out of every five women have some type of cardiovascular disease, which accounts for 48 percent of all deaths in the United States. This annual death rate is ten times greater than that reported for breast cancer.[53] Forty-five percent of women can expect to develop coronary disease in their lifetime; 30 percent of those will die from it. An additional 10 percent will die from a stroke. Yet women rate cancer as a greater health concern by more than a two-to-one margin.[54]
- *Osteoporosis.* Incidence increases with age, and nearly 80 percent of osteoporosis sufferers are women.[55] Osteoporosis affects 50 percent of women over age forty-five and 90 percent of those over age seventy-five. Each year, the disease contributes to 1.5 million bone fractures of the hip, spine, and wrist.[56] By the year 2015, twenty-five million women will be affected. Fractures due to osteoporosis cost the U.S. health care system more than $10 billion annually.[57] An estimated fifty thousand Americans die annually from complications of osteoporosis-related hip fractures.[58]
- *Breast cancer.* The leading cause of death among women aged forty to fifty-five, breast cancer is the most common form of cancer in U.S. women and kills 44,300 of them annually, with more than 184,000 new cases diagnosed each year.[57] Approximately 75 percent of women diagnosed with advanced breast cancer are post-menopausal.[58]
- *Ovarian cancer.* Most commonly occurring in women in their fifties, it is estimated that approximately twenty-six thousand new cases of ovarian cancer are diagnosed each year. About one in seventy women will develop ovarian cancer during their lifetime; about 14,500 will die each year due to it.[59]
- *Migraine.* Eighteen million women suffer from migraines, contrasted to 5.6 million men.[60]

Exhibit 1.1.   Conditions Affecting Women.

measures and treatment for health problems that can occur in the early and prime reproductive years (see Exhibit 1.2). Too often, therefore, they act on none of these concerns. This increases their risk, especially of eating disorders and smoking.

Women in this life segment are most vulnerable to eating disorders; 90 percent of all people with threatening eating disorders are adolescent and young adult women. Of the more than one million Americans battling bulimia, women are the vast majority.[24]

Women under age twenty-three make up the fastest-growing sector of smokers in America.[25] What will this mean to the health care

Adolescence and Early Adulthood (Ages 15–21):
Building the Foundation for a Healthy Lifestyle

Educational Needs
   Self-esteem and body image
   Building relationships
   Coping with peer pressure
   Accepting self-responsibility
   Proper diet
   Regular exercise
   Good posture
   Hair and skin care
   Understanding tobacco, drugs, and alcohol
   Understanding sexuality
   Preventing sexually transmitted diseases
   Understanding and using (when and if needed)
      contraception
   Knowing automobile safety
   "Buying in" to family values
   Understanding the psychology of family dynamics
   Defining and achieving educational goals
   Setting career goals

Medical Needs
   Rubella immunization (if necessary)
   Contraception
   Pregnancy counseling
   Prenatal care
   Recognizing physical and psychological problems
   Premenstrual syndrome (PMS)
   Menstrual irregularities
   Eating disorders
   Addiction
   Persistent acne
   Asthma
   Vaginal discharge
   Sexually transmitted diseases (STDs)
   Attention deficit disorder
   Social acting-out
   Social withdrawal
   Suicidal thoughts

Prime Reproductive Years (Ages 22–35):
Developing and Maintaining a Healthy Lifestyle

Educational Needs
   Reinforcing the elements of a healthy lifestyle
   Forming lasting relationships
   Career building
   Family building
   Sexual satisfaction
   Family relationships
   Financial planning
   Time management

Exhibit 1.2.   Early and Prime Reproductive Years.

Medical Needs
    Hepatitis B immunization (if required)
    Conception, prenatal care, and obstetrical delivery
    Contraception
    Pregnancy counseling
    Annual screening
    Cervical cytology
    Urinalysis
    Baseline screening
    Mammogram (age 35)
    Recognizing physical and psychological problems
    Infertility
    Abnormal Pap smear
    Benign breast disease
    Irregular reproductive cycles
    Abnormal body weight
    Dysuria
    Congenital heart disease
    Stress
    Anxiety
    Frigidity, anorgasmia
    Poor interpersonal relationships

Exhibit 1.2.   (*Continued*)

Source: Copyright © 1998 by G. William Bates. Used with permission.

industry twenty or thirty years from now? According to the American Cancer Society, women might have a 20 to 70 percent higher risk of developing lung cancer than men by then. Extrapolating from the last few years' data shows that the outlook is not promising. In 1998, lung cancer was expected to kill 23,000 more women than breast cancer. Each year, more than 140,000 women die of lung cancer and other smoking related diseases.[26]

The Thirties

In their thirties, many women experience the sometimes overwhelming pressures of work, children, and home. Juggling these can have health consequences if they ignore their own health while attending to the needs of others. Generally, they do not become seriously ill as a result, but often they start to notice natural changes in body shape and skin texture. This spurs many women to pursue health prevention, typically through exercise, diet, and skin care.

Also, more women have babies in their thirties now than in earlier generations; the first-birth rate among this group has nearly tripled since 1975.[27]

The Forties

By their forties, most women have developed a sense of self and a career, and most have already given birth. Some of these women, many with young children, find that it is difficult to find time for self-caring. Unless single, the forties are not a me-first period in a woman's life, but they realize they still have a chance to change or start a new career. However, many feel that their life is half over and they have accomplished nothing for themselves.

Most women in their forties want to safeguard and enhance their health, they become aware that health maintenance is harder, and they don't bounce back as easily. They also worry about the cosmetic effects of aging; the biggest visible skin change for women takes place around the age of forty-five. Also at this age, women begin to worry more about breast cancer. And they begin to experience more ailments (see Exhibit 1.3), such as gastrointestinal problems (up to 25 percent of Caucasian women and 80 percent of African-Americans and Asians develop some degree of milk intolerance, for example). Women also become more prone to irritable bowel syndrome, and about 40 percent in this age group have some degree of stress incontinence. The risk of gallstones increases as well, with 20 percent of women developing them as a result of excessive fat consumption, obesity, or high estrogen levels from previous pregnancies. The forties are also a time for vision change, especially the loss of near vision.[28]

The Fifties

In their fifties, many women are settled in a career, have raised their children, and have much insight and experience. Most also enter menopause at this state, and that physical change can often cause great psychological change (see Exhibit 1.4). Many feel their mortality, and they begin to focus on taking care of themselves and enjoying life. Some embrace and celebrate middle age, others undergo a rebirth, a new beginning. Others are not so positive.

Depression occurs in all life span segments, but women in their fifties often scrutinize themselves harshly and feel bad about what they think is missing in their life. Whatever her outlook, a healthy fifty-year-old woman today still has over a third of her life to look forward to.

A woman's metabolism slows down in her fifties, and her health risks really start to increase. It is not uncommon for them to be overweight, gaining two to five pounds per year.[29] According to the National

Completing Reproduction and Preparing for Menopause (Ages 36–45)

Educational Needs
  Reinforcing the importance of a healthy lifestyle
  Nutritional counseling and weight management
  Establishing or reinforcing an exercise program
  Smoking cessation (if a smoker)
  Preventing osteoporosis
  Avoiding excessive ultraviolet-ray exposure
  Self-esteem
  Healthy body image
  Nurturing the spirit
  Finding relaxation responses
  Stress management
  Sexual satisfaction
  Family relationships
  Adjusting to adolescent children and aging parents
  Meeting financial goals and objectives
  Meeting career objectives
  Introducing hormone replacement

Medical Needs
  Completion of reproduction
  Achieving first pregnancy (if deferred)
  Achieving final pregnancies (if more children are desired)
  Ensuring contraception
  Sterilization (either partner)
  Annual screening
  Breast examination
  Cervical cytology
  Hematocrit
  Urinalysis
  Periodic screening
  Mammography
  Bone densitometry (if risk factors apply)
  Gonadotropins (if early menopausal symptoms)
  Androgens (if loss of libido)
  Recognizing physical and psychological problems
  Premenstrual syndrome
  Dysfunctional uterine bleeding
  Uterine leiomyoma
  Urinary stress incontinence
  Pigmented nevi and other skin lesions
  Joint symptoms
  Dyspnea (if smoker)
  Addiction

Exhibit 1.3.   Late Reproductive Years and Perimenopause.

Source: Copyright © 1998 by G. William Bates. Used with permission.

Making the Transition from Reproduction (Ages 46–55)

Educational Needs
> Reinforcing healthy lifestyle
> Self-esteem
> Healthy body image
> Family relationships
> Helping children complete education, establish careers and families
> Helping parents deal with challenges of aging
> Aligning partnership goals with mate
> Sexual satisfaction
> Evaluation and maintenance of career goals
> Securing financial future

Medical Needs
> Contraception
> Hormone replacement
> Early detection of physical and psychological problems
> Annual screening
> Mammogram
> Hematocrit
> Urinalysis
> Stool occult blood examination
> Dental evaluation
> Periodic screening
> Hearing (if there is auditory deficiency)
> Bone densitometry (if risk factors apply)
> Differentiated cholesterol (if family history of coronary artery disease)
> Androgens (if history of loss of libido)
> Colonoscopy (if risk factors for colon cancer apply)
> Tonometry (if risk factors for glaucoma apply)
> Visual acuity (when symptoms of presbyopia occur)
> Recognizing physical and psychological problems
> Dyspareunia
> Dysfunctional uterine and postmenopausal bleeding
> Loss of libido (male and female)
> Hot flushes
> Joint pain and deformities
> Back pain
> Pigmented nevi and other skin lesions
> Dyspnea and easy fatigue
> Urinary incontinence
> Dyspepsia
> Constipation
> Sleep dysfunction
> Mood volatility
> Short-term memory loss
> Depression

Exhibit 1.4. Perimenopausal and Early Menopausal Years.

Source: Copyright © 1998 by G. William Bates. Used with permission.

Center for Health Statistics, 52 percent of women between fifty and fifty-nine were overweight between 1988 and 1991. The fear of losing their sexual attractiveness may also become a real concern; some women, looking back rather than forward, deal with these feelings by altering their bodies to fit the cultural stereotype. Some go from personal trainer to dermatologist to plastic surgeon on a never-ending quest for their lost youth.[30]

The Sixties

Of all age segments, this one may be the most critical (see Exhibit 1.5). This is when many women start to really feel old. It is a very common age for facelifts, for example. The major issues for women in their sixties are retirement or changes in involvement at work, losing a spouse, shifting family responsibilities, physical decline, chronic illness, and changes in appearance. Each can lead to a decrease in social interaction, a very important part of life.

By this time many women must decide about therapies for hormone replacement, osteoporosis, or breast cancer. Lesser disorders such as incontinence and sexual dysfunction are also of concern, and their eyes, ears, and teeth also need regular care.[31]

Turning sixty is not so bad. Older women today are healthier than in the past. One reason is that many health care providers now emphasize preventative health care, living a healthy life, and being part of the health process.[32]

The Seventies Plus

Not long ago, the idea of health after seventy seemed almost unthinkable. No real thought was given to providing information about diet, exercise, and sexuality to women that old. But now many such women are healthy, active, living independently, and participating in family, community, and social life.

More and more women in their seventies function as women in their fifties did a couple of decades ago.[33] Still, about three-fourths of people over seventy-five who live in nursing homes are women.[34] Women of that age are likely to be widows (64 percent), and the majority live alone. Of women eighty-five or older who live alone, the poverty rate is 32 percent, more than twice the rate for other women and men (15.2 percent) in this age group (see Exhibit 1.6).[35]

Maximizing the Attainments of Life (Ages 56–65)

Women who reach age 65 will, on average, live for another nineteen years.

Educational Needs
    Reinforce the ways to maximize good physical and mental health
    Understand the physical changes of aging
    Implement dietary supplement program
    Strengthen partnership with mate
    Secure retirement income
    Reevaluate career goals
    Solidify family relationships
    Develop latent interests
    Shift the balance of work and play
    Begin the transition from career to retirement

Medical Needs
    Medical needs become more complex and comprehensive at this stage. Women
    should follow the recommendations of their primary care physician. This is a
    time to maximize sound nutrition, regular exercise, safety, and intellectual
    stimulation—now and for the remainder of life.

Exhibit 1.5.   Mature Adulthood.

Source: Copyright © 1998 by G. William Bates. Used with permission. Life
expectancy data from B. Ettinger, "Guidelines for Established Osteoporosis
Treatment," *Menopause Management,* 1997, 6(5), 6–9.

Still, reaching this age can be very emotionally and physically challenging, and even lonely. Most women over eighty today have fewer
children than their earlier counterparts, and these children are likely
to be in their sixties or older and to face some impairments of their
own.[36] Also, such women may have to confront the stress of caring for
an ailing spouse, grief and loneliness over loss, changing self-image
over new physical limitations, and worry over Alzheimer's disease
(which affects two to three times more women than men).[37] All this
can lead to depression.

FITNESS AND HEALTH THROUGH THE DECADES

A significant part of the health care equation throughout life is a matter of fitness and exercise. Considering that women are usually the
gatekeepers of health care, it is important to recognize their own fitness goals and needs throughout the life cycle.

Over the past two decades, our society has placed an increasing
value on staying fit and healthy. Early on, some would say, the main

The Retirement Decade (Ages 66–75):
Enjoying the Fruits of Labor and Years Ahead

Women who reach age 75 will, on average, live another twelve years.

Educational Needs
  Profit from mistakes made
  Remember the outstanding moments of one's life
  Enjoy retirement
  Realize the most important things in life
  Appreciate the importance of grandchildren and try to encourage and support
    them
  Continue exercise

Advanced Age (Ages 76–85): Enjoying Each Year and Coping with Loss

Women who reach age 80 will, on average, live another 8.9 years. Those who reach 85 will, on average, live another 6.4 years.

Educational Needs
  Accept the fact that there will be more medical problems
  Walk daily
  Eat nutritionally
  Stay on prescribed medication and take regularly
  Continue interest in reading and television
  Maintain contact with friends
  Stay in touch with grandchildren
  Be grateful for years past
  Strengthen spiritual life

Exhibit 1.6.   Retirement and Advanced Age.

Source: Copyright © 1998 by G. William Bates. Used with permission. Written by Susan Hill Rayburn; life expectancy data from B. Ettinger, "Guidelines for Established Osteoporosis Treatment," *Menopause Management,* 1997, 6(5), 6–9.

message to women was to look as young possible for as long as possible. That message persists, no doubt, but today the culture also stresses the health benefits of exercise. Thus reasons for exercising are changing, especially for women.

More women now exercise out of habit and to maintain health, rather than just to improve appearance. A survey found that females in every age group over age twelve, as of 1996, are more involved in fitness than males in any age group. It also revealed that women between eighteen and twenty-four are the most active exercisers, with more than 27 percent exercising at least a hundred times per year, and that the second most active age group among women are those between forty-five and fifty-four, of whom 25 percent exercise frequently.[38]

Female exercise also translates into an enormous amount of buying power—women buy 40 percent of all sports equipment.[39] One market research firm reported that in 1993, women purchased 94 percent of all step-aerobics equipment, 70 percent of all stair climbers, and 65 percent of all treadmills.[40]

The increased awareness of health benefits gained through exercise is recognized by women of several generations and will have a significant impact on women's health in the long term as well as on the health care services they will demand. It is, for many women, a type of insurance against illness, and an aspect of care providers would be wise to consider.

WOMEN'S HEALTH INSURANCE

In most states, individual health insurance policies cost women between the ages of fifteen and forty-four double what they cost men, and on average health care costs are 45 percent higher for working women than for working men.[41] Regardless of where they live and how well they seem to do as a group, women are still affected by some factors more often then men. One is poverty: more than 70 percent of the 1.3 billion people living in poverty are women.[42] In the United States, African-American women over the age of seventy-five are the poorest group of elderly people (43 percent of the total), followed by Hispanic women of the same age (30.1 percent), according to 1992 figures from the U.S. General Accounting Office. Overall, black women experience triple the rate of poverty of white women and are also slightly less likely to be insured.[43] Is it likely that the women who desire more frequent physician visits are at or near the poverty level? With the link between poverty and ill health well established in professional literature, the extra physician visits these women wish to make are probably preventive or of minor severity in nature, but their economic condition and health plans leave them with no real choice but to wait until their health is much worse. The result is greater cost to them, their health plans, and in many cases to the provider. Obviously, the feminization of poverty is a very real social and business issue that cannot be overlooked.

Managed care is the major player in women's health care, with the coverage rate nearly double that of fee-for-service programs.[44] How do the one-sixth of women who want more medical care fit into this equation? One could assume that most of them are customers of managed care plans. What advantage could there be for any payor to limit physician visits? It might show a short-term financial benefit but risks financial disaster in the long term. Even though the health care industry's move toward managed care and toward better health through prevention and early intervention is generally considered a good thing, many health care plans, both managed care and fee-for-service, still have old paradigms to overcome.

Consider the issue of birth control. The five most commonly used reversible methods of contraception are the Pill, IUDs, diaphragms, Norplant, and Depo-Provera injections. Only 39 percent of HMOs cover all of these methods.[45] Condoms aren't covered by most health insurance plans either, maybe because they are not prescriptive. If insurers were to forgo $16 extra per enrollee per year (the cost of covering contraceptive supplies and services), they could save between $9,000 and $15,000 per woman in pregnancy-related expenses over five years, according to a recent study in the *American Journal of Public Health*.[46] Of the 97 percent of large-company fee-for-service plans covering prescription drugs in general, only 33 percent pay for birth control pills, and 49 percent of traditional fee-for-service plans cover no contraception at all.[47] Contraception may be the largest out-of-pocket health-related expense for young women, who are probably the group least able to afford it. Yet contraception presents an enormous opportunity for health care plans. Providing customers with preventive services can make good financial sense and increase a plan's value to its customers.

In the future, insurers may have to explain why women in their reproductive years pay double for their individual health insurance policies. Women pay an average of 68 percent more in out-of-pocket health expenses than men do, as many basic reproductive health services aren't covered by insurers, according to the Women's Research and Education Institute.[48] On the surface, it seems payors are trying to realize short-term savings by truncating treatments uniquely required by women without exploring other options—such as paying for contraceptives, thus saving money in the long term and increasing a plan's attractiveness to customers.

SUMMARY

This chapter looks at women as a component of the population, as an economic force, and as gatekeepers and consumers of health care. These factors show that women are the leading health care customers.

Women have sounded a wake-up call, and the health care industry's initial response has been a shift of research money and design care devoted to products for women. This is good, but much more needs to be done if near-future health care demands are to be adequately met.

Due in part to our country's declining birth rate, soon older people will outnumber children. This will have profound effects on the delivery and use of health care services, pension systems, family life, medical research agendas, end-of-life decisions, private and public resource allocation, and living arrangements. To prepare, links between acute and long-term care services, the two pillars of comprehensive geriatrics, need to be made. Although family women are still primary caregivers, their ability to care for older people has changed. More women work outside the home today, yet even as they continue to care for their children, older family members increasingly need help at the same time. This, coupled with women's longevity and decreasing birthrate, will result in a significant increase in the number of elderly women in need of expanded services. Therefore, the expansion of hospital services, nursing homes, and community-based services, as well as assisted living, are necessary to serve our aging population.

To win in the women's health care marketplace—to be able to truly listen, hear, and fulfill—one must understand in depth the many concerns and changes that women face throughout life. Health care providers who can position themselves now to meet the needs of women from adolescence to old age are those who are able to build a continuum of care that allows them to retain women as customers for life. That's a market-share strategy with true longevity.

Notes

1. Butler, R. N. "Population Aging and Health." *British Medical Journal,* 1997, *315,* 1082.
2. Butler, "Population Aging and Health."
3. U.S. Bureau of the Census. *We the American Women.* Washington, D.C.: U.S. Department of Commerce, Economics and Statistics Administration, 1993.
4. U.S. Bureau of the Census. *We the American Elderly.* Washington, D.C.: U.S. Department of Commerce, Economics and Statistics Administration, 1993.
5. "Trends That Will Affect Retail Pharmacy." *Chain Drug Review,* Apr. 27, 1998, p. Rx12.
6. U.S. Bureau of the Census, *We the American Women.*
7. "Trends That Will Affect Retail Pharmacy."

8. Heller, A. "Women's Health: Tackling the Critical Issues." *Drug Store News,* Sept. 22, 1997, p. CP11.

9. "Industry Sees Power in Women's Health Issues." *Indianapolis Star and News,* June 19, 1998.

10. Cannon, C. M. "The Business of Women's Health." *Working Woman,* Mar. 1998, p. 37.

11. "Anthem Blue Cross and Blue Shield Launches Tri-State Women's Health Program." *PR Newswire,* June 19, 1998, p. 619.

12. "Anthem Blue Cross and Blue Shield."

13. "Anthem Blue Cross and Blue Shield."

14. "Anthem Blue Cross and Blue Shield."

15. Cannon, "The Business of Women's Health."

16. "Reaching Women, Health Gatekeepers." *Healthcare PR & Marketing News,* May 14, 1998.

17. "Anthem Blue Cross and Blue Shield."

18. "Offer Women Health Care Decision Makers High-Quality Service." *About Women & Marketing,* Oct. 1997, p. 10.

19. Liebmann-Smith, J. "The Hot Doctor Debate." *American Health for Women.* July-Aug. 1997, p. 28.

20. "Reaching Women, Health Gatekeepers."

21. Cool, L. C. "Forgotten Women: How Minorities Are Underserved by Our Health Care System." *American Health for Women,* May 1997.

22. Cool, "Forgotten Women."

23. Cool, "Forgotten Women."

24. "Women's Health: On the Road to Discovery, Part II." *Med Ad News,* Jan. 1997.

25. "Society for the Advancement of Women's Health Research Calls for Ban on Tobacco Advertising Targeted at Women." *PR Newswire,* Apr. 23, 1998.

26. "Society for the Advancement of Women's Health Research."

27. Gleason, S. "In Your 30s." *Town & Country,* Oct. 1997, p. 204.

28. Guernsey, D. "In Your 40s." *Town & Country,* Oct. 1997, p. 208.

29. Laurence, L. "In Your 50s." *Town & Country,* Oct. 1997, p. 214.

30. Laurence, "In Your 50s."

31. Behbehani, M. "In Your 60s." *Town & Country,* Oct. 1997, p. 222.

32. Weinhouse, B. "In Your 70s and Beyond." *Town & Country,* Oct. 1997, p. 228.

33. Weinhouse, "In Your 70s and Beyond."

34. Cannon, "The Business of Women's Health."

35. Gonyea, J. G. "Age-Based Policies and the Oldest-Old." *Generations,* Fall 1995, p. 25.

36. Gonyea, "Age-Based Policies."
37. Kyriakos, T. "Women's Health Issues Move Toward the Forefront of Science." *Drug Store News,* Mar. 16, 1998, p. 9.
38. Johnson, D. "Tracking Fitness: From Fashion Fad to Health Trend." *Futurist,* May 1998, p. 8.
39. Smith, W. K. "Tapping Women's Buying Power." *Boating Industry,* Jan. 1996, p. 25.
40. Dogar, R. "Sweat Equity: Women Exercise Buying Power." *Working Woman,* Mar. 1995, p. 16.
41. Gorman, M. O. "Show Me the Coverage: Why Women Pay More for Less Health Insurance." *American Health for Women,* Nov. 1997, p. 37.
42. Craft, N. "Women's Health Is a Global Issue." *British Medical Journal,* 1997, *315,* 1154.
43. Cool, "Forgotten Women."
44. "The *Glamour*/Eckerd Study Eyes Women's Health Issues." *Chain Drug Review,* Nov. 3, 1997.
45. Gorman, "Show Me the Coverage," p. 38.
46. Gorman, "Show Me the Coverage," p. 38.
47. "Five-State Study Shows Disturbing Gaps in Contraceptive Coverage." *Medical Utilization Management,* Oct. 15, 1998.
48. Gorman, "Show Me the Coverage," p. 37.
49. Mincieli, G. "Women's Health: On the Road to Discovery, Part I." *Med Ad News,* Jan. 1997, p. 1.
50. "Anthem Blue Cross and Blue Shield."
51. "Anthem Blue Cross and Blue Shield."
52. Mincieli, "Women's Health."
53. Kyriakos, "Women's Health Issues."
54. "Speakers at Women's Health Symposium Say Cardiovascular Disease Is Number One Killer of Women." *PR Newswire,* Feb. 13, 1998.
55. Cannon, "The Business of Women's Health."
56. Mincieli, "Women's Health."
57. "Anthem Blue Cross and Blue Shield."
58. Mincieli, "Women's Health."
59. Mincieli, "Women's Health."
60. Kyriakos, "Women's Health Issues."

CHAPTER TWO

The Women's Health Movement

Genie James

———≈≈≈———

To succeed in the women's health care marketplace, it helps greatly to understand the genesis and transformation of women's health issues. That makes it possible to predict how the women's health movement will continue to evolve, and to anticipate and prepare for how it will influence the future of the health care industry.

Men and women may have been created equal, but they certainly were not created the same. In the clinical arena, this notion has been expanded and validated through gender-specific disease studies. Gender difference has also led to a wave of pop psychology discussions—*Men Are from Mars, Women Are from Venus*,[1] for example. Lay people often follow the women's health movement through other such public forums. For example, over the past two decades, breast cancer, once spoken of only behind closed doors, has become a favorite topic of those campaigning for public office. Constituents—and their mothers, daughters, and sisters—are all affected one way or another.

The women's health movement has reached a critical mass. Developing a proactive women's health strategy must now be considered mandatory for care providers who want to succeed in the future. But this is not a matter of having an OB floor, pink walls, and baby bill-

	Age					
	Under 45		45–64		Over 65	
Condition	Men	Women	Men	Women	Men	Women
Arthritis	25.8	35.8	204.9	289.7	374.5	538.4
Hypertension	38.1	32.3	221.9	215.1	291.7	424.3
Sinusitis	99.9	127.7	162.7	199.5	136.9	162.3
Orthopedic deformity	92.4	98.2	151.4	170.8	141.5	197.9
Hearing impairment	49.7	29.6	197.8	106.0	395.5	269.1
Heart disease	27.3	34.2	137.4	101.5	320.4	263.5
Migraine	20.9	23.9	23.9	87.3	3.3	33.6
Varicose veins	4.8	25.8	17.6	73.6	38.7	99.2
Hemorrhoids	22.7	28.9	71.1	70.8	46.2	68.1
Thyroid disease	2.0	12.2	9.5	44.9	10.8	45.0
Cataracts	1.2	2.5	17.4	26.3	98.0	193.8
Anemia	4.6	25.9	2.5	22.5	9.5	29.5

Table 2.1.   Incidence of Twelve Chronic Conditions per 1,000 Population, 1993.

Source: National Center for Health Statistics.

year to primary care physicians than males.[12] Beyond this, according to one report, women make 75 percent (some put it at 80 to 90 percent) of consumer health care decisions.[13] When it comes to influencing market share, women are customers worth cultivating.[14]

Later chapters in this book discuss other aspects of women's health as a managed care strategy. Here, however, is a description of some of the more readily apparent questions, issues, and concerns with respect to women's medicine, biopsychosocial care, health management, and Medicare.

Women's Medicine

Given that women are not like men, how should their differences and preferences be factored into the design of a continuum of care? Some women contend that sex differences are important and complicated enough to warrant a new specialty analogous to pediatrics or geriatrics. "We're not talking about lady doctors delivering medical care to lady patients," says Eileen Hoffman, codirector of the women's health program at Mount Sinai Medical Center in New York. "We're talking about an art and science that's focused on the female."[15]

But how do you develop a more relational and patient-sensitive plan for women's health services when company reengineering is going on? When government reimbursement is being cut? When full-time employees are being reduced?

Biopsychosocial Care

If women want to be treated as whole persons, their providers and care-givers must offer a balanced-body biopsychosocial approach to health and well-being. This is a collaborative model for care that includes physical and mental health professionals as well as the family.[16]

Many health systems are experimenting with mind-body-spirit ap-proaches. But how many do so in a way that fits with aggressive inte-gration strategies and revenue targets? The ideas of prevention and wellness appear to have gained momentum over the past few decades. But aren't health care systems still in the business of taking care of sick patients? Where do wellness and prevention fit in? "Women want re-spect; they want choices; they want preventive care," says health care consultant Sally Rynne. "That's what women have clamored for." And the intent today, she says, is to get people to take care of themselves because it is cost-effective.[17]

Even when health care CEOs agree with mind-body-spirit ap-proaches and that prevention and well care are important, they often don't have the resources to developing a new model of care, nor the budget to hire consultants to advise how to accomplish such an ideal. More often they have to figure out how to deliver quality care for less money and with fewer people. Also, despite the looming impact of capitation, CEOs still spend more time developing strategies to put sick people in hospital beds rather than to keep them healthy and on the street.

In July 1998, Hillary Rodham Clinton returned to the site of the first Women's Rights convention. To a crowd of about sixteen thou-sand, she pointedly stated an agenda for advancing the women's health movement: greater pay equity for women, universal health care cov-erage, expanded child care aid, and a tougher stand against domestic violence. If she is on target, and many women across the nation seem to think she is, then health care systems that want to be successful in the future have to decide how to weave those themes into their char-ter. But how?

First of all, does focusing on disease and treatment miss the point? "It's easier to prescribe a pill than to address the precarious economic status of women," says Judith G. Gonyea, professor of social work at Boston University who specializes in women and aging. "People's health is about their housing, their nutrition, about feeling socially connected, which all may have a much greater bearing on their physical health status than their level of estrogen does." In research especially, the line between science and politics has been tested in the debate over whether women have been shortchanged.[18] Again, the question emerges: How can a health care system keep a balance between its financial objectives and public policy mandates?

There is a reason why baby boomers are sometimes called the sandwich generation. Women who delay motherhood quite often simultaneously raise families and care for aging parents. Infant health, adolescent health, and elder care services—not to mention personal time management and work-family stress—are all real issues to the female market segment that most health systems are trying to court. Developing a women's health strategy is not just a matter of expanding and improving an OB unit or building a breast health center. Is it possible to develop and implement a strategy that addresses all women's health concerns throughout life?

Health Management and Medicare

What is the relationship between the demographics of female baby boomers, their health management, and a Medicare strategy? The federal Balanced Budget Act of 1997 cut spending for Medicare capitated plans by about 9 percent over five years by limiting growth to that below the growth in traditional Medicare fee-for-service plans, reducing geographic variation, and removing the teaching payment included in the capitated payment. In many cases, that dramatically alters the competitiveness of capitated plans compared to Medicare fee-for-service plans. As a result, capitated plans will be better off in some places and worse off in others.[18]

The new Medicare reimbursement scenario could put providers in a position where they have little or no incentive to provide more than minimal services, apply new technology, or encourage the use of new (more expensive?) drugs. Medicare does now pay for more preventive services, but providers certainly wouldn't be motivated to expand them to include theme preventive services not covered or other loss-leaders such as lifestyle management. All health care systems try to make decisions in the best interest of patients, but if making a right decision hurts providers financially—if it costs them money to lose money—what can they do? As Medicare services become managed care, where will mission statements, quality care, consumer demand, patient satisfaction, and revenue streams intersect? If women are the majority of its patients, how does a health system ensure that it is the chosen provider? If risk makes the healthier population most desirable, how does disease management work for the chronic concerns that women suffer as they age?

SUMMARY

This chapter addresses the impact of feminism on women's health care, changes in the women's health movement since the 1850s, and trends for the next millennium. It discusses how that movement will continue to affect the delivery of services. Providers must examine each women's health care issue according to its mission, business objectives, and local market forces. How these are prioritized and addressed should depend on the competition, hot issues, and the availability of manpower, systems, and capital. The health care system that succeeds in the new millennium knows that handling women's health care well will capture customers and retain revenue.

Notes

1. Gray, J. *Men Are from Mars, Women Are from Venus.* New York: HarperCollins, 1992.
2. Goodman, E. "When Women Stood Up at Seneca Falls." *St. Louis Post Dispatch,* July 20, 1998, p. B7.
3. Aburdene, P., and Naisbitt, J. *Megatrends for Women: From Liberation to Leadership.* New York: Fawcett Columbine, 1992, p. ix.
4. Bellafonte, G. "Feminism: It's All About Me." *Time,* June 29, 1998, p. 58.
5. Covey, A. (ed.). *A Century of Women.* Based on a documentary script by A. Jacoba with H. Schulman and K. Thompson. Atlanta: TBS Books, 1994, pp. 71–73.
6. Blumenthal, S. J., and Wood, S. F. "Women's Health Care: Federal Initiatives, Policies and Directions." In S. Gallant, G. Puryear Kieta,

and R. Royak-Schaler (eds.), *Health Care for Women.* Washington, D.C.: American Psychological Association, 1997, p. 3.

7. Ferriman, A. "NHS, 1948–1998: Free Reign Women's Health." *Guardian,* July 1, 1998, p. 12.

8. Boston Women's Health Book Collective. *Our Bodies, Ourselves.* Boston: Boston Women's Health Book Collective, 1971.

9. Blumenthal and Wood, "Women's Health Care."

10. Crose, R. *Healthcare for Women.* Washington, D.C.: American Psychological Association, 1997, pp. 221–222.

11. Rosvold-Brenholtz, H. *National Women's Health Report,* Vol. 19, No. 1. Washington, D.C.: National Women's Health Resource Center, 1997, pp. 1–6.

12. James, G. *Making Managed Care Work: Strategies for Local Market Dominance.* Burr Ridge, Ill.: Irwin, 1997, pp. 158–159.

13. Aburdene and Naisbitt, *Megatrends for Women.*

14. Mansnerus, L. "More Research, More Profits, More Conflict." *New York Times,* June 22, 1997. Women's Health Special Edition, p. 3.

15. James, *Making Managed Care Work,* p. 177.

16. Mansnerus, "More Research," p. 4.

17. Mansnerus, "More Research," p. 2.

18. Rodgers, J. *Congress Reforms Medicare Capitated Payments: How Will It Affect Managed Care Plans?* New York: Price Waterhouse LLP, 1998.

CHAPTER THREE

Consumer Pressure Meets Public Policy

Genie James

————

T his chapter considers how public policy and legislative action define women's health issues. *Public policy* here refers to government mandates that, in general, tell health providers what they should do, can do, and how things ought to be done. *Politics* means the making and influencing of public policy, but not necessarily its administration.

For the past decade, policymakers have fluctuated in their preference between government intervention and managed care. Because neither model has succeeded in controlling costs, a new consumer-controlled model is now being touted as the practical answer to the health care cost dilemma.

Health care decision makers should follow the trends in their market just as they would if they had their own money invested in the stock market. Women's health issues can be just as volatile as stocks and, if monitored closely, just as telling in a health system's final market share.

Women now have the critical mass needed to push their health agendas in the policy and political arenas. The drivers of reform are beginning to realize that women's health services wield clout with both voters and the powers that control the health care dollar. Women are a force to be reckoned with at the federal, state, and local levels. The trends speak for themselves.

A PUBLIC POLICY PERSPECTIVE

Most agree that public policy on health should benefit everybody, help prevent illness, and educate the population. But when it comes to turning words into action, the agreement disappears. The variety of services and how they are organized varies greatly from one locality to another. The trend seems to be that contemporary public policy is determined less by what public health professionals know how to do than by what the political system in a given area decides to do.[1] If that seems cynical, just consider what has occurred with both Medicaid and Medicare in the past few years.

In the early 1990s, some thought that the only way to deliver health care sensibly was to return to a public policy approach: move away from the competitive market dynamic, where hospitals duplicate services and technology in an attempt to get their share of the market, and toward a scenario where hospitals determine their product and service mix based on needs and gaps in the continuum of care in the communities they serve. This seemed to be common sense, especially given the rumblings about managed care that were beginning at the time and the shrinking reimbursement trends that were already being evidenced in California.

Then the health care system was flush with profit from sick care. Public policy principles were not in vogue, because they brought no profit. Consequently, no one was paying to develop expertise in public policy perspectives. This was not good news, particularly for consultants or for the long term.

In 1994, the *Quality Letter for Healthcare Leaders* championed a "return to the public health principle." It described a burgeoning new wave of community health initiatives across the country, and stated: "In part, these efforts reflect the rediscovery of a basic public health principle, enunciated two decades ago by visionaries such as Henrik Blum, M.D., professor emeritus at the University of California–Berkeley School of Public Health. Dr. Blum counseled students that health and well-being not only are products of medical care, but are also 'closely linked' with community factors such as financial resources, health manpower, socio-economic status, education and housing."[2]

Why is a public policy emphasis on health and well-being now re-emerging? Because the governments and employers that have been paying the bills are going broke. Managed care is often accused of being merely a way to control costs, but its basic intent is to shift the health care industry from one where the cash register rings every time someone is sick to one that makes money even if a patient never walks in the door. As James F. Fries has said, "By emphasizing both disease prevention and individual responsibility, we can reduce yearly health care costs by $200 billion."[3] But accomplishing that requires a paradigm shift.

First with managed care and then with changes in Medicare and Medicaid reimbursement, health care providers have been burdened with a need to deliver care for less, even as disease prevention and individual responsibility have not picked up the slack. Most likely, public policy will increasingly demand that providers take joint responsibility for the covered lives in the communities they serve. The Balanced Budget Act and the new reality of Medicare risk are evidence that there is no turning back. True enough, but what makes this important in the context of women's health?

REDEFINING HEALTH

A lasting legacy of the women's health movement is a renewed emphasis on the need to develop a much broader definition of health. Regina Herzlinger says that good health care includes easy access to it.[4] An analysis of 803 families, for example, found that single-parent families need care but fail to obtain it more often than two-parent families. Other studies found that children in single-parent families receive fewer preventive and other health care services than those in two-parent families. The lack of social support in single-parent families likely influenced these results. More women in the single-parent families reported that "fewer than two persons [were] available for help in times of need." Indeed, inconvenience is probably one reason for the puzzling failure of many well-intentioned efforts to improve the health care of children in single-parent families and the rates of immunization of poor urban infants.

Herzlinger describes instances in which well-intentioned health care activists offered free services in the hope of alleviating the cost barriers for such services as immunizations, vaccinations, and screenings. An intensive analysis of cost and utilization revealed a surprise:

convenience was more important than cost. Lower-income won
are more likely to be paid by the hour and, therefore, do not want t
give up wages even for health advantages. To this target population, it
is more important to focus on the tangible—bread on the table and
money in the pocket—than a more abstract concept of disease prevention.

In today's environment, when a health system is faced with an access issue such as the one Herzlinger describes, the discussion often
leads to a debate about the health system's role in community health
initiatives.

PROVIDERS TAKE A PUBLIC HEALTH
FOCUS

As an example, consider domestic violence, one of the most prevalent
problems in society today and one that demands a public health focus
and a new kind of commitment from health care providers. In the
1970s, the United States criminal justice system woke up to the problem of domestic violence. Since then, women's advocates and policy-
makers nationwide have been pushing the health care system to focus
on domestic violence as a public health problem that sends thousands
of women to hospital emergency rooms each year. The damage caused
by domestic violence does not show up just behind closed doors, in
the privacy of someone's home. It shows up on the hospital's balance
sheet because of its tie to preventable emergency room utilization.

Advocates and policymakers have succeeded in making an impact:
in 1994, the American Medical Association issued diagnostic and
treatment guidelines on domestic violence, finding the problem so
prevalent that doctors should routinely and directly ask all women
about abuse—not just in emergency rooms but in primary care, prenatal clinics, and other health settings. In 1995, California became the
first state to require all hospitals and clinics to develop procedures for
screening patients to detect domestic violence.[5]

According to Debbie Lee, associate director of the Family Violence
Prevention Fund in San Francisco, close to four million women are
physically abused each year, and many seek help in a medical setting.
One study of an urban emergency room found that 30 percent of
female trauma victims had been battered. According to the Federal
Bureau of Investigation, 30 percent of homicides of women were at the
hands of their husbands or boyfriends. And a study at Rush Medical

..ter in Chicago found that the average charge for medical services כ abused women, children, and older people was $1,633 per person per year, a total of $857.3 million a year. Preventing the need for these people to go to emergency rooms in the first place is clearly a great way for providers to cut costs while improving health care.

Health care providers are in a unique position to intervene in cases of domestic violence, given the recurring health problems and frequency of visits by battered women to health care facilities. Indeed, women look to their providers as a place to get information on domestic violence. Most women don't want to go to the police or the courts, but all see doctors at some point.[6] Since 1992, the Joint Commission for the Accreditation of Healthcare Organizations has required that accredited emergency departments have policies and procedures with respect to domestic violence and a plan for educating staff on the treatment of abused adults. As a result, many health care institutions have developed assessment forms for domestic abuse.[7]

Shifts in reimbursement are causing health systems to reexamine and embrace a public policy perspective. The American Hospital Association reports that the large majority of hospitals now have some form of community health initiative in place. Most hospitals and health systems emphasize health and well-being in their mission statements. Some do better than others at translating vision into action. Because women make most health care decisions for their families, any effort to put a new public health principle into action will fail unless women believe it adds value to their and their family's life. So a new policy must be socially conscious and reflect surging consumer demand (see Exhibit 3.1).

WOMEN'S POLITICAL CLOUT

Lobbyists for women's groups have proven over the past decade that women can demand more than better infant car seats. Now it is clear that women vote for politicians who provide the dollars, political clout, and results needed to satisfy their health care needs. Today, an army of special interest groups lobby Congress on women's behalf.

In 1990, the National Institutes of Health (NIH) established the Office of Research on Women's Health to set goals and policies for women's health research and help women get their fair share of attention in clinical research. Vivian Pinn says its $10 million budget funds studies on women "that might not otherwise be done."[8] The under-

- Health services for women must be designed to meet the needs of the "whole woman": mind, body, spirit, and connection to community.
- They must move beyond a focus on reproductive health and meet the needs of women throughout life.
- Access, convenience, education, information, and relationship-centered care must be the framework of health services delivery.
- Ethnicity and cultural differences should be factors.
- Meeting the needs of women requires addressing their socioeconomic concerns.
- Access to up-to-date and appropriate health information for female clients is very important.
- Research and data collection methods must be developed for women's health.
- The rights of women to choice, confidentiality, and informed consent are paramount.
- A holistic approach across a continuum of care is mandatory. Fragmentation of services is no longer acceptable.
- Women want wellness and health promotion.
- Local markets need specific programs to meet the needs of the women who live there.

Exhibit 3.1.   Principles for Women's Health Service.

standing that biomedical research has historically focused more on the health problems of men is one reason this special office was created. Five state governments now have their own offices. In 1991, Congress passed the Women's Health Equity Act, a twenty-two–bill package ensuring federal funding for research on women's health issues.[9]

The NIH Revitalization Act of 1993 provided legislative language to mandate the Office of Research on Women's Health (ORWH). One of the first actions undertaken by ORWH was to establish an agenda for women's health research that included the entire life span, and to better define gender differences and similarities. The ORWH agenda encompasses issues that go far beyond women's reproductive capacity, cutting across and integrating scientific disciplines, medical specialties, psychosocial and behavioral factors, and environmental determinants in a multidisciplinary and collaborative approach. It addresses sex and gender perspectives of women's health, as well as differences among special populations of women. The agenda encompasses the entire life span of women, from birth through adolescence, reproductive years, menopausal years, and the elderly years. Included are studies to better define normal development, physiology, and aging in women. The agenda includes conditions that are unique to women, as well as those that affect both men and women.[10]

Not one woman sat on the appropriations subcommittee that oversees NIH when the campaign to increase funding for women's health research began. In 1997, four women sat on that subcommittee. Funding for women's health research continues to face the same financial constraints as other areas of domestic spending, but now at least women's health advocates are at the table when the decisions are made.[11] The ORWH, which now has a $14 million annual budget, encourages researchers and health care practitioners to address women's unique needs, and the Food and Drug Administration today demands solid evidence that new drugs are effective and safe for women before it approves them. Pharmaceutical companies and financial analysts are also convinced that companies can profit from meeting the health needs of females. For instance, heart medicines specifically designed for women are being developed and marketed.[12]

Congress has definitely taken note. The committees that develop the health research budget have studded their reports in recent years with demands for more research on disorders that predominantly affect women. The allotment for women's health in the 1999 budget of the Department of Health and Human Services, which covers most federally financed research, is $2.3 billion, up 30 percent in three years.

Great strides are being made. And consider how much greater they might be. There is still a dearth of women in politics: 50 percent of the population is women, but twenty-six states had no women in the 105th Congress. Only nine out of one hundred Senators, and fifty-four of the 435 representatives in the House, are women.[13]

A great impact of the 105th Congress in 1998 was the passage of several pieces of legislation, one on the treatment of breast cancer and another on childbirth. The Women's Health and Cancer Rights Act stipulates that any health plan that provides medical benefits for mastectomy must also provide coverage for breast reconstruction for patients who want it. Another new law says that group health plans and insurers generally may not restrict the length of hospital care for childbirth for either mother or child to less than forty-eight hours following vaginal delivery or ninety-six following a cesarean, with certain exceptions.

Another big consumer issue was evidenced by the legislative tug-of-war over a 1998 bill requiring most health insurance plans for federal workers to cover prescription contraceptives. Some lawmakers pushed for its passage, but it eventually was dropped, perhaps because it was tagged by many who favor the right to abortion. But should women pay full price for birth control pills while men can pick up Viagra for a $5 co-pay? Never mind that the cost of covering contraceptives is far below the cost of caring for unwanted babies.

Women's health issues are indeed bringing public policy directives and political agendas together. The result should be the linking of human and health services delivery to foster better health care. But in many markets such collaboration reduces revenue for providers. Unless, of course, they realize that the market is driven by consumers, understand that women's health is much more than a matter of gender-specific disease, and realize that success involves gaining market share, earning revenue, and being socially conscious. To do that requires understanding how much influence and buying power women wield.

WOMEN AS HEALTH CARE CONSUMERS

When health system executives begin to understand the buying power of women, many jump to the conclusion that they should immediately build a shiny new women's center complete with a cosmetic surgery salon, a weight management specialist, and an aquarium (for the aesthetics). That might work in some places, but not in most. What do women in your area want? In most cases, they want the basics, not the extras.

Marjean Coddon, vice president of the Learning Institute of Quorum Health Resources, Inc., in several conversations with the author distilled all the rules into their most critical features:

- *Access and convenience:* Women want themselves and their family members to be able to see a doctor when it works for them, even if it's nights or weekends. They don't want to wait more than fifteen minutes. They don't want to fuss with parking. They want to be able to find their doctor's office without a road map for the labyrinth of offices in a modern medical building.

- *Education and information:* Women want to know all options for treatment, including nontraditional and complementary therapies. They want to know, objectively, how good your organization and your doctors are so they can pick you or somebody else to provide their care. In time, standardized comparative outcome and performance profiles may be commonplace, published by several sources—your organization, competitors, accreditors, buyers, and information clearing houses.

- *Sensitivity of providers:* Women want care givers who listen. Because managed-care physicians often are pushed to see more and more patients in less and less time, many of their patients feel like objects on an assembly line. Providing relationship-centered care is the key to success for health care systems; they must satisfy patients even as they are operationally efficient.

Today, the path to consumer orientation is blocked by internal obstacles. Tomorrow, leaders will commit to building consumer-oriented organizations. That will require investments in people, products, services, and infrastructure—and astute investors will reap the rewards. Organizations will build competitive advantage by recognizing that consumerism is a wave they can ride to higher customer satisfaction and volume, market share, and economic performance. Good leaders will force their organizations to serve consumer desires better and to develop faster and better techniques for measuring those desires.[14]

DETERMINING AND IMPROVING CONSUMER SATISFACTION

What do you do if you are in a competitive marketplace and the patient satisfaction results aren't in yet? Many health systems are betting that an increased emphasis on community health collaborations will help them cover their bases on both public policy issues and women's consumer demands. Some CEOs personally handle five to ten patient complaint calls per week just to keep their fingers on the pulse of the real issues. Others walk the halls at night and talk to a few awake patients and family members to find out how they are really doing. Dick Davidson, president of the American Hospital Association, recommends another approach: "Poor public perception is our biggest problem because it directly affects our resources. Last year, Congress was able to balance the budget on the backs of hospitals because they know the public didn't care what happened to us. There's a challenge here for trustees. Our ability to change the public's perception rests with them. It's a combination of management and governance, but the buck stops at the boardroom."[15]

One innovative approach to determining patient satisfaction has been developed by the Health Communication Research Institute, Inc. (HCRI), a nonprofit organization headquartered in Sacramento, California. The product, called Patients First, uses the "patient experience" to evaluate health care services and user-friendly prepaid phone cards for high response rates. The patient uses the phone card to call an automated service that records his or her satisfaction with all levels of care received; as a bonus the patients receive twenty to thirty minutes of free long-distance service for their own use. Questions asked of the patient can be changed at any time. "Use of prepaid phone cards in other types of marketing research has proven effective. People are motivated to respond to questions when they can receive free long distance service in return," says Marlene von Friederichs–Fitzwater, executive director at HCRI. "People are also inclined to be more honest in responding to an automated service rather than to a person."[16]

Consumers are making noise about the current health care system's poor responsiveness. Congress is legislating in response. As a result, there is now a revolution on the public policy front.[17]

Consumers are upset about managed care—and the medical provider community has a responsibility to help them through the quagmire. An underlying theme of some legislation, including the Patients' Bill of Rights, is the need for patients to understand their choices and to make informed decisions regarding their care. Education and information are key and can be used to build competitive advantage. For instance, once you have achieved demonstrably superior performance, disseminate outcome and performance facts through marketing and advertising. If you also educate consumers to use and interpret the data properly, your advantage increases.[18] Take it a step further:

- What if you were to create an internal function for professional patient advocacy that simply helped consumers understand their choices in this managed care world?
- What if you created and distributed a glossary of managed care terms?
- What if you had a telephone line dedicated to helping consumers understand their health plan's coverage, benefits, and billing?
- What if you positioned your organization as the consumer's ally by helping your consumers manage their managed care, helping

them understand which plan will cover their anticipated health and wellness concerns, what drugs and alternative therapies are covered or not, and what their rights are?

These extra steps might provide ways for your hospital, health system, or physician group to be viewed as the hero—and develop a competitive edge.

SUMMARY

Developing a competitive advantage may not be easy. It requires constant assessment of consumer needs—and acknowledgment of the role of women in health issues. The pivotal points will be enhanced convenience, knowledge transfer, and customer intimacy. Because of the ubiquitous nature of perceived sensitivity and relationship building, health systems will need some hard data to assess how they are doing along the way. Hospitals, health systems, physicians, and augmentative care providers all face the same challenge. Everyone is being asked to do more with less and to make sure that it still meets the customer's demands while offering that personal touch.

Notes

1. Marczynski-Music, K. K. *Health Care Solutions: Designing Community-Based Systems That Work.* San Francisco: Jossey-Bass, 1994, p. 118.
2. *Quality Letter for Healthcare Leaders,* June 1994.
3. "Community Health: Catalyst or Catastrophe?" Presentation at Quorum Health Resources, 1996.
4. Herzlinger, R. *Market Driven Health Care: Who Wins, Who Loses in the Transformation of America's Largest Service Industry.* Reading, Mass.: Perseus Books, 1997, p. 24.
5. Lewin, T. "Seeking a Public Health Solution for a Problem That Starts at Home." *New York Times,* June 22, 1997, Women's Health Special Edition, pp. 1–2.
6. "Domestic Violence: Why Don't Providers Ask?" *NAPWH Focus,* 1998, 2(2), 2, 8.
7. Satel, S. L. "There Is No Women's Health Crisis." *National Affairs,* Winter 1998, p. 21.

8. Pinn, V. W. "The Role of the NIH's Office of Research on Women's Health." *Academic Medicine,* 1994, *69.*

9. Grundy, C., and others. "Women's Health Legislation in the 105th Congress." *Women's Policy,* 1998, 3.

10. Legato, M. J. "Research on the Biology of Women Will Improve Healthcare for Men, Too." *Chronicle of Higher Education,* May 15, 1998.

11. Stein, B. "We've Come a Long Way, Baby, but the Road Is Long." *Nashville Tennessean,* Sept. 30, 1998, p. 2E.

12. Peters, T. *The Circle of Innovation: You Can't Shrink Your Way to Greatness.* New York: Knopf, 1997, pp. 395–411.

13. Press, C. *Consumerism in Health Care: New Voices.* New York: KPMG, 1998, pp. 1–2, 20–24.

14. Grayson, M. "An Interview with Dick Davidson." *Hospitals and Health Networks,* July 5, 1998, p. 14.

15. Grayson, "Interview with Dick Davidson."

16. von Friederichs–Fitzwater, M., personal conversation.

17. Grayson, "Interview with Dick Davidson."

18. Press, *Consumerism in Health Care,* p. 20.

CHAPTER FOUR

Following Women's Dollars

Genie James

———~~~———

This chapter shows how women are an economic force to be reckoned with. Their buying power and political clout make a female-targeted strategy essential for any provider system accelerating into the next millennium.

WOMEN FLEX FINANCIAL MUSCLE

By the year 2008, women aged forty-five to sixty-four will be the largest and richest segment of the U.S. population—the first time in history that the largest demographic will also be the wealthiest. What's more, much of that wealth will not be inherited from husbands and relatives as in the past, but earned by women themselves.[1]

How has this come about? Two primary variables contribute to this dramatic variation from the traditional image of women as mother and wife—and one who, if she worked outside the home, did so to bring in a second paycheck to cover those little extras and luxuries. First, there are simply more women. Consider these facts:[2]

- Half of all marriages end in divorce.
- A majority of women outlive men.
- A growing segment of women choose to remain single.
- More women are in the workforce.

Education is the second variable. For the first time, females aged twenty-five to twenty-nine have pulled ahead of their male counterparts in educational achievement. The annual report on educational attainment says 88.9 percent of women in that age group had a high school diploma, compared with 85.8 percent of men. And 29.3 percent of women earned an undergraduate college degree or higher, compared with 26.3 percent of men. It "indicates a dramatic improvement by women, who historically have been less educated," says Jennifer Day, author of the report. More education translates to better-paying jobs.[3]

Women are not just getting their degrees; they are moving steadily into the entrepreneurial ranks, increasing their impact on global markets, and positioning themselves to be even bigger players in the next century, according to participants in the fifth Global Summit of Women.[4]

According to a survey conducted by the National Foundation for Women Business Owners, women continue to form new businesses at roughly twice the national average. Though the chance to pursue their entrepreneurial dreams was cited as the main reason for this, 51 percent of the women surveyed said they were frustrated with the lack of flexibility in corporate America, and 44 percent cited their failure to advance. When asked what it would take to lure them back to corporate America, 58 percent of women answered "nothing," 24 percent said "more money," and 11 percent said "more flexibility."[5] The findings should be a wake-up call for corporate America.

What all this means is that women, as a whole, have more money in a world where money still means power. Because women are not satisfied with how the male-dominated work place has been run, they are leaving old-style corporations and defining for themselves a better way of running business—and it is working. Many women are highly successful financially in this new world order. Poverty continues to be a very real concern facing too many citizens, particularly women and children, but some light has begun to shine at the end of the tunnel.

WOMEN'S HEALTH DOLLARS

Health systems now have a choice: capitalize on the economic power and intellectual capital in the hands of female customers or continue business as usual. For the health system trying to position itself for the millennium, the latter is probably not a sustainable option. Health system decision makers, physician leaders, and board members are wise to ask the following questions:

- If women are driving so many health care decisions—for themselves and their families—how can we tailor our managed care strategy and consumer education programs to reach them?

- If there truly is a feminization of poverty in this nation, how can our health system help address this issue?

- If women have increasingly more disposable income, what retail strategy can help us tap into this potential revenue stream?

Health systems must choose which retail strategies and product niches to pursue. The choices must take women into account. For example, as women age, progress in the corporate world, and have more disposable income, their desire to improve their appearance will coincide with their desire to maintain and improve health. One niche that holds promise is cosmetic surgery. Echelon Health, Inc., a physician practice management (PPM) company based in Brentwood, Tennessee, manages the business side of practice for plastic and reconstructive surgeons. Cheryl Carlson, president and chief executive officer of Echelon, says, "Cosmetic surgery services represent an anomaly in health care, creating a highly competitive market. The demand of elective procedures is growing and not greatly influenced by managed care. Cosmetic surgery is one of several attractive private-pay niches."

Carlson adds, "The baby boomers are a definite factor in the business potential in cosmetic surgery. Plastic surgery is attractive to aging baby boomers . . . as a potential help in their personal and professional lives and because of their attitudes toward personal health, anti-aging and self-improvement."[6]

The data support her: forty percent of all people who elect to have cosmetic surgery are between the ages of thirty-five and fifty, and women are 88 percent of them.

WALL STREET'S LESSONS

If your organization needs convincing that the female customer is emerging as a whole new subset of the economy, perhaps it can learn from the players on Wall Street.

It's not easy to pinpoint how or even when the business of women's health attained its new financial status. One watershed came in 1996, when Smith Barney hired Melissa Wilmouth, an analyst with a background in medical supplies and technology. Her mission was to identify hot stocks of small companies that produce medical devices. Wilmouth found that several new companies producing women's health devices or procedures had gone public. Many of these firms were subsequently bought out by medical industry giants. Wilmouth compared notes with Anne Malone, a Smith Barney analyst who specializes in large medical device firms. After two months of research, they identified a new arena for investment: companies specializing in women's health.[7]

Wilmoth was a keynote speaker at the National Association for Women's Health (NAWH) 1998 conference. She said, "On Wall Street, demographics times dollars equals [investor] demand." A few examples follow to test her equation.

U.S. drug companies are booming. Recent earnings reports show double-digit growth—in some cases more than 30 percent. Why are they doing so well? Demographics. An aging population is increasing the demand for pharmaceuticals and medical devices. Note that most of these older people are women.[8]

Female baby boomers are reaching menopause at a rate of more than two thousand per day. As they enter menopause, some develop disorders that can be treated with pharmaceuticals. This is reshaping the pharmaceutical industry. Women account for more than 51 percent of the population and are a major influence on consumer spending and marketing plans. Hoping to satisfy them, pharmaceutical executives are redesigning their pipelines and marketing strategies. In 1997, there were more than three hundred drugs in development to treat female-specific diseases and conditions.[9]

Factor the demographics and the demand with the fact that women now have more disposable income, and you can see why Wall Street analysts anticipate spectacular bottom-line results from both the pharmaceutical and medical device industry segments.

So far, the investments appear to be paying off. The market for drugs that treat female-specific diseases and conditions has been growing at a compound rate of 18.8 percent since 1990. (See Exhibit 4.1.) The market for women's drugs was valued in 1998 at about $5.7 billion. Market analysts estimate it will exceed $10.6 billion by 2000.[10]

The dollars drug companies are earning in women's health should emphasize the importance of the women's market and give health system executives an idea about new strategic partnerships. (For further discussion, see Chapter Thirteen.)

NICHE PLAYERS TAKE MARKET SHARE

Another presentation at the NAWH 1998 conference, given by Kathy Hanold, addressed the importance of hospitals and health systems learning the lessons from Wall Street in order to seize opportunity. Hanold listed many compelling reasons for changing approaches, including declining revenues, fewer in-patient cases, reduced access to capital, risks of physician defection, and increasing employer and payor expectations. As discussed further in Chapter Six, Hanold believes that new market entrants (for-profit niche players and investor-owned companies) will serve as true catalysts in driving market competition. It follows that targeting women's health is a logical strategy that has already led to success for Health South in the area of episodic injury and MedCath in the area of cardiac concerns. New entrants already succeed—Medisphere Health Partners in Tennessee, Renaissance IntegraMed in Texas, and Mid-South Health Alliance in Virginia, for example.

Hanold went on to say that capitalizing on the expanding women's health market requires concentrating on the creation of competitive advantages via operational excellence, product leadership, and customer intimacy. The risk of doing nothing is much greater than the risk of deciding to shut down an OB unit, for example. By not attending to female consumers as change agents for product and service design, hospitals and health systems jeopardize both revenue and market share.

What do the women in your market want? Don't bank on them to choose your facility just because they gave birth there ten or twenty years ago. Instead, learn exactly what services women want and how they want them delivered. Customer intimacy means more than ensuring that

- *Menopause.* Demand: Worldwide, the total hormone replacement therapy market is estimated at $1.9 billion. Market Response: There are nine major estrogen replacement therapies on the market that help control menopausal symptoms. Sample/Projected Earnings: Estrin, which was approved in April 1996, was expected to earn $40 million in 1997.
- *Depression.* Demand: Women experience depression at more than twice the rate of men; 7 percent of women will suffer major depression in their lifetime, compared with 2.6 percent of men. Market Response: Numerous prescription medications belong to this group. Sample/Projected Earnings: Prozac remains Lilly's biggest selling drug and the leader in the antidepressant category with sales of $2.4 billion in 1996.
- *Osteoporosis.* Demand: An estimated 20 million American women have osteoporosis. The cost for treating the disorder is about $10 billion to the U.S. health care system annually. Each year, this disease is the cause of 1.5 million bone fractures of the hip, spine, and wrist. About one in four women are at risk of developing osteoporosis. Market Response: If drug therapy is indicated, women can choose from four major products. Sample/Projected Earnings: Merck's Fosamax was expected to have 1996 sales of $235 million.
- *Breast Cancer.* Demand: This most common form of cancer in the U.S. kills 44,300 American women a year. Market Response: In 1997, ten major products specifically indicated for the treatment of breast cancer were on the market. Sample/Projected Earnings: One product on the market, Taxol, was originally discovered during a plant-screening program sponsored by the National Cancer Institute. It generated sales of $815 million in 1996. The cost of therapy for one person is $3,199.22 (Ovarian Carcinoma Solution 30mg/5ml, 0.25/day, 365 days).
- *Ovarian Cancer.* Demand: Accounts for 18 percent of all gynecological neoplasms or abnormal growth of tissues, most commonly occurring in women in their 50s. It is estimated that about 26,000 new cases of ovarian cancer are diagnosed each year. About one in 70 women will develop ovarian cancer during their lifetime. About 14,500 deaths result each year. Market Response: There are seven major products on the market to treat ovarian cancer. Sample/Projected Earnings: One of these products, Paraplatin, generated estimated sales of $375 million in 1996.
- *Migraine.* Demand: Migraine is much more common in women than men; 18 million women suffer from migraine compared with 5.6 million men. Market Response: There are nine major products on the market, classified in two categories: beta blockers and ergot derivatives. Sample/Projected Earnings: Imitrex is the only migraine therapy that treats the multiple symptoms of migraine. Financial analysts estimate the 1996 worldwide sales of Imitrex were $775 million.
- *Cervical Cancer.* Demand: About 15,700 American women, 450,000 cases worldwide, are diagnosed with cervical cancer each year. Market Response: Thin prep pap smears.
- *Morning Sickness.* Demand: In the U.S., 50,000 pregnant women are hospitalized each year due to nausea and vomiting associated with the first trimester of pregnancy. Market Response: The market for pregnant women has proven to be risky, making pharmaceutical companies reluctant to enter.

Exhibit 4.1. Conditions Affecting Women: Sample Market Responses and Earnings.

Source: Mincieli, G. "Women's Health: On the Road to Discovery, Part I." *Med Ad News,* Jan. 1997, p. 1.

female patients have a pleasant experience when inside your doors; it means knowing how to get them inside to begin with.

Cheryl E. Stone, senior vice president of Rynne Marketing Group in Evanston, Illinois, stresses the importance of primary market research that gathers qualitative information first: "This helps identify existing gaps in care from the women's perspective. For instance, a community may have the appropriate ratio of mammography services to population, but your focus groups may tell you they would like to have mammograms done before they go to work. In this case, the lack of available mammography services between 6:30 and 8:30 A.M. is a gap in care."[11]

Stone also emphasizes proper depth of data and comprehensive interpretation of market research: "Critical variables such as percentage of managed care penetration, sociodemographic mix, competitive forces, geographical access, and provider willingness must all be aligned before one can hope to take an idea and translate it into success. Too often a decision is made to develop a program or add a service because a key decision maker read an article or attended a seminar where innovative success stories were shared. Garnering new ideas and learning from others should be applauded if the ideas are critically examined to reveal their affinity with the local market situation."[12]

DEMOGRAPHICS, DOLLARS, AND CONSUMER DEMAND

Building on Wilmoth's equation for success on Wall Street, the health system's equation for long-term viability will be demographics times dollars times consumer demand equals product and service design and delivery. The following methodology can be helpful in moving from concept to strategy.

First, analyze your demographics. Chances are that women compose a high percentage of the population you serve. Also, examine the breakout of women's cohorts and profile the unique concerns associated with each. This can provide hard data regarding age-based needs for the female customer. Factor in women's impact on purchasing and choice decisions (that is, how often women thirty to sixty years old make health care decisions for other family members).

Second, profile your payor mix according to what they cover for women's care. More women today have their own insurance, and in most markets they have more disposable income. Make sure you understand how managed care could affect utilization of your services, but also take a new look at what women may be willing to pay for out-of-pocket.

Third, find out what your customers want and how they want it delivered. In essence, hospitals and health systems must learn to respond to informed and selective consumers or they won't have a business to worry about. In today's health care industry, only the fit will survive. Becoming fit requires responding to consumer demand with flexibility, agility, and sensitivity—all in the context of cost-efficient operations.

SUMMARY

Women are the gatekeepers of health care utilization and they use health care more often than men, beginning from the time of their first gynecological exam to the time when they become the decision makers who purchase health care for their families, and on through their later years.

This chapter emphasizes that women wield influence over purchasing decisions—and they control the dollars. This is true not only of the woman on the street but the woman who chairs a health system's financial review committee. Can the health care industry demonstrate a willingness and ability to reinvent itself for a female consumer-driven future?

Notes

1. Stein, B. "Numbers, Money Bring Women Power." *Nashville Tennessean,* May 13, 1998, p. 1E.
2. Tevis, C. "Farm Women Flex Financial Muscle." *Successful Farming,* 1998, 6, 58.
3. Manning, A. "Women Outpacing Men by Degrees." *USA Today,* June 29, 1998, p. 2B.
4. Lederer, E. M. "Women Now a Major Force in Global Market." *Nashville Tennessean,* July 25, 1998, pp. 2A, 11A.
5. "Female Entrepreneurs Shun Corporate America." *Nashville Tennessean,* Oct. 17, 1999, p. 5A.
6. Cannon, C. M. "The Business of Women's Health." *Working Woman,* Mar. 1998, p. 38.

7. Meyers, B. "Drugmakers Have Healthy Outlook." *USA Today,* July 20, 1998, p. 1B.
8. Mincieli, G. "Women's Health: On the Road to Discovery, Part I." *Med Ad News,* Jan. 1997, p. 1.
9. Mincieli, "Women's Health."
10. Mincieli, "Women's Health."
11. Stone, C. E., personal conversation.
12. Stone, personal conversation.

CHAPTER FIVE

Adapting Product Lines and Information Technology for the Consumer

Genie James

One of the greatest criticisms of health care over the past decade is that it has left the patient out of the equation. Now it seems that to reinvent the industry requires looking beyond patient care to consumer power. What does this mean for the hospital and health system of the new millennium? Many of today's strong new voices are calling for a total revolution of the health care sector.

How does one begin this major overhaul and translate an industry-wide revolution down to local operations? In part it may be as simple as asking people in the community what they want and how they want it delivered. Because women make most health care purchasing decisions, savvy providers will question many women and reconsider how they market to them. They will be innovative in developing new ways to learn what women want. This chapter discusses the importance of market intelligence—understanding the needs, motivations, and issues your customers face in order to earn the right to ask for their business.

UNDERSTANDING AND SERVING YOUR CUSTOMER

What do women want from their health care providers? As we've seen, they want the following:

• Access and convenience

• Information and education

• Sensitivity from their care givers

• A mind-body-spirit approach that treats patients as more than symptoms

They want these features for their personal care as well as the care of their family and their community.

Imagine one place where women can attend to all their basic health needs. In this place, all the regular screens for yearly physicals are performed by professionals who have undergone extra training in women's health. There is an emphasis on wellness and prevention as well as a commitment to teaching women about their own health care. There is also a commitment to getting people in and out without delays—even on a one-hour lunch break. There are evening and weekend hours, and child care is an option.[1]

Not every community needs a full-fledged mini-mall concept for women's health. To know which ones do requires asking questions and listening to the answers. In May 1997, *Self* magazine set out to profile the top ten women's care hospitals in America. It found that many health care organizations are paying attention and have already begun to develop strategies to target female consumers. Those that demonstrate both market share retention or growth and new sources of revenue have one predominant characteristic—they listen to their customers. Sounds simple, but the notion of first defining your target customer base, learning clearly what the customer wants, and, finally, designing a business model for cost-effective product and service delivery too often gets skewed between negotiating managed care contracts and entering into network agreements. A list of possible women's wants gleaned from the *Self* survey appears in Exhibit 5.1.

It's worth noting that convenience and access are two of the most important features that a woman considers when choosing a provider. These tend to run neck-and-neck with the patient's perception of her care giver's sensitivity to her needs, thus underscoring the importance of communication with patients.

Have target customers rank by checking the appropriate number, 1 being least important and 5 being most important.	1	2	3	4	5
A place of its own					
One-stop shopping					
State-of-the-art technology					
Wellness facilities					
Continuing community education					
Specialized counselors on staff					
Alternative therapies					
Pregnancy-related services					
Screening and treatment for sexually transmitted diseases					
Providers with experience or training in women's health					
Doctor-patient discussions					
Female physicians and staff					
Domestic abuse services					
Strong managerial direction					
Convenience					
Written statement of philosophy					

Exhibit 5.1.   What Do Women Want from a Women's Health Center?

Source: Adapted by Kim Walker, former director managed care and marketing for PrincipalCare, Inc., from Korn, P. "America's 10 Best Hospitals for Women's Care." *Self,* May 1997, p. 187.

The model that is developed in the local market should reflect how women's health fits with the overall mission and vision of an organization. In December 1997, a new Center of Excellence in Women's Health—with a broad mission of improving the health of Tennessee's 2.6 million women—was proposed for the University of Tennessee in Memphis. If created and funded, the $4.9 million center is intended to carry out the mission of the institution through research, education, service delivery, and outreach programs statewide. Its list of objectives includes efforts to screen and detect breast, cervical, and uterine cancer, and osteoporosis among women with less access to health care, reducing teen pregnancy and domestic violence, and increasing prenatal care.[2]

The projected budget made more than a few people nervous. But if your mission and vision emphasizes relationships and healing, it is hard to limit the price. Not every hospital will have—or want—a facility complete with a massage room and a waterfall, but all should aspire to have an atmosphere where a kind word and a smile are the signature of the organization.

Much as managed care has narrowed the price window between competing facilities, and even as provider panels have helped, consumer choice remains important. The health system executive must understand what motivates an end user to pick one health plan over another. As a recent Kaiser Family Foundation study (see Chapter One) showed, nearly 98 percent of the women surveyed agree that it's important for a health plan to provide high-quality health care. Access is also perceived to be important. When presented with a hypothetical situation in which their health plans were discontinued and they had to choose another, 99.2 percent agreed it would be very important to know how easy a potential plan made it to get the care they needed.

Women do not want to pay more for less health care. In most states, individual health insurance policies cost women between the ages of fifteen and forty-four about double what they cost men, according to Steven Miles, an associate professor of medicine and geriatrics at the University of Minnesota Center for Bioethics in Minneapolis. The insurers' reasoning: these women might get pregnant and require expensive maternity care. Yet the Washington-based Women's Research and Education Institute has reported that during their reproductive years, women pay an average of 68 percent more in out-of-pocket health expenses than men do, because many basic reproductive health services aren't covered by insurers.[3] According to a study sponsored by the Alan Guttmacher Institute, 21 percent of managed care organizations surveyed in five states offer little or no contraceptive coverage out of a misplaced concern about costs, and more than half of the plans neglect to inform recipients of whether they provide the coverage. Only one in four have involved family planning agencies in their networks. Rachel Gold, a researcher with the family planning research and advocacy organization, says basic contraceptive care would cost employers about $17 per employee per year, less than the cost of a one-month supply of birth control pills. The cost savings come from preventing pregnancies.[4]

Preventive care is also high on women's list of concerns. Most (96 percent) agree it would be at least somewhat important to know how well a prospective plan keeps its members as healthy as possible.

PRODUCT LINES AND PREVENTIVE MEDICINE

Nutritional therapy makes an attractive product line in the prevention category but it is also critical to chronic disease management, which is so important in keeping health plans financially healthy. Nan Allison, of Allison and Beck Nutrition Consultants, Inc., in Nashville, Tennessee, has provided statistics regarding nutritional therapy's role in disease management.

The chronic conditions listed by the National Women's Health Initiative—osteoporosis, hypertension, cardiovascular disease, diabetes, breast cancer, and obesity—all have nutrition as a primary and critical component to prevention and treatment. In fact, diet is the first step in established treatment protocols for four of these conditions: cardiovascular disease, obesity, diabetes, and osteoporosis.

Osteoporosis affects more than twenty-five million women over the age of forty-five. Only one-quarter to one-half of women with hip fractures ever regain previous levels of functioning; 20 percent need extensive medical attention. In the United States, annual costs associated with osteoporosis care and rehabilitation are estimated at $10 billion.

Hormone replacement therapy is an effective prevention tool in early postmenopausal years. But the best way to prevent osteoporosis is to build strong bones early in life, not just with calcium but with magnesium and boron (both found in fruits and vegetables), low intakes of caffeine, alcohol, and sodium, and avoidance of excessive protein.

Hypertension is also more problematic for women than men. Moderate weight reduction (if overweight) and a low sodium diet are the first steps in treatment.

Cardiovascular disease, including coronary heart disease and stroke, is the number one cause of illness and death in North American women. One of two will die of some cardiovascular event. Dietary treatment with a low-fat, high-fiber, weight-loss (if overweight), low-sodium food plan is the first step in the treatment protocol for heart disease—prior to introducing medication.

Diabetes is the number six cause of mortality for women in America.[5] *Diabetes mellitus* ("sweet diabetes") can start suddenly, or it can be silent for weeks or months after it begins. In this disease, the body finds it difficult to use sugar, so it accumulates in the blood. Blood sugar levels are thus high, and organs such as the eyes, kidneys, and small arteries all over the body are gradually damaged. There are several varieties of diabetes mellitus in women:[6]

- *Juvenile (Type I) Diabetes:* This variety of diabetes may start in children or young adults, almost always before the age of forty.
- *Diabetes During Pregnancy:* Diabetes is often diagnosed during pregnancy.
- *Adult-Onset (Type II) Diabetes, or Non-Insulin-Dependent Diabetes Mellitus (NIDDM):* This form of diabetes usually develops in overweight people over the age of thirty who have diabetes in their family.

Breast cancer will affect one of nine women in North America. Diet may make the difference between the progression or prevention of the disease. Emerging data show that body weight, dietary fat, fruit and vegetable consumption, phytochemicals, and antioxidants all play a role. Certain breast cancers are more responsive to specific dietary therapies.

Obesity ranks second to smoking as a cause of preventable death in the United States. Approximately one-third of North American women are overweight, up from 25 percent in the 1970s. There is a weight-gaining trend despite women's preoccupation with body weight and despite the massive effort and billions of dollars spent to control weight and eat reduced-calorie foods. Well-designed, clinically sound programs that help to educate and that lead to modification of detrimental behaviors can effectively show an organization's concern for the general health and well-being of its patients. These can also be critical ways to retain customers that a provider is at risk of losing—especially where keeping them healthy is tantamount to financial survival.

Weight loss and weight management programs are other potential product lines. Approximately 95 percent of those suffering from anorexia or bulimia are women. Adolescent girls are particularly vulnerable to eating disorders. Health plans would do well to strongly consider obesity and weight control if they are to meet the expectations of most women.

Randy Killian, executive vice president of the National Association of Managed Care Physicians, emphasized the point that managed care plans cannot afford to ignore the importance of nutritional therapy: "We who have been working in the managed care environment believe that the future is going to be health promotion, disease prevention, treating illness and maintaining wellness. Nutrition is going to be a tremendous part of everything we do in the future."[7]

HEALTH MANAGEMENT *IS* MANAGED CARE

According to the Kaiser Family Foundation study about what women desire in their health plans, catching health problems at an early stage was close to the top, with 99 percent judging it either important or very important. With regard to health plans in general, large percentages of women feel that keeping costs of coverage low (95 percent) and having a wide range of doctors (92 percent) is important, but the percentage rating these as very important is not as high as it is for other factors. In keeping with this, only one in five (19 percent) rank a wide choice of doctors as their most important selection criteria, and only 17 percent cite keeping costs low.

When it comes to finding out about health plans, women trust friends the most. As the majority of them are probably not clinically trained, it would stand to reason that the friends are passing on not quality ratings but their own experience with the provider. At any rate, studies indicate that most women (94 percent) view friends and relatives as a believable source of health care information; half credit them as being very believable. Recommendations from individual doctors are not welcomed with quite as much enthusiasm. Although 93 percent find them believable, six in ten see them as only somewhat believable.[8]

The trends are there. Just as we saw with the health system, women are looking to their managed care plans to help to keep them well (see Exhibit 5.2). They want flexible health plans whose providers have extended hours and convenient locations. What it means to serve the customers needs to be evaluated. And, as providers begin to move away from a sick-care industry, health management and preventive medicine will emerge and differentiate tomorrow's viable leaders across the health care industry.

INFORMATION TECHNOLOGY: POWER FOR CONSUMERS

Physicians were once heralded as the all-knowing members of our culture. What happened? It is almost as if Toto has pulled back the curtain to reveal that the one we thought was the all-powerful Oz—our physician—is simply a normal person. Information technology is our Toto. That is, the information age has put great volumes of medical information at the fingertips of the average consumer. The Internet empowers anyone with access to a computer with reams of data about disease, treatment options, and self-help. If clinical knowledge has been the cloak of power, then it no longer shrouds only our physicians. Thanks to information technology, the physician and the patient stand as two people in the same room.

Certainly the years of intensive training that any physician has gone through maintain their merit. Physicians and nurses and scores of augmentative providers have extensive training and expertise that will continue to play a significant role in the care of patients. Still, who is more vested than the individual when it comes to keeping themselves and their families healthy? The consumer really is the most seminal provider of care, and now that consumer has access to screens and screens of data to parlay into a care plan for themselves and their families.

Few topics have received as much hype and publicity as the Internet and related technology. Even Intel chairman Andrew Grove proclaimed in a *Newsweek* interview that workers in almost every industry, including health care, should view the Internet as a "tidal

Top 10 HMOs: Factors Cited in High Rankings

- Pays for prescription contraceptives
- Covers breast reconstruction after mastectomy
- Lets a women self-refer to an OB/GYN
- Has short (three- to five-day) wait time to schedule a routine office visit
- Provides follow-up care after hospitalization
- Funds research
- Provides patient education and outreach activities to its members (such as twenty-four-hour hotlines)
- Provides products and services for wellness and disease prevention
- Provides access to emergency care
- Has short customer service wait times
- Covers some complementary medicine (chiropractic, acupuncture, naturopathy)
- Provides health care and wellness education (print and programs)
- Provides special support for managing chronic conditions
- Has good policies and rates for screening and immunizations

Exhibit 5.2.   What Women Want from Their Health Plans.

Source: Extrapolated from Korn, P. "The 10 Best HMOs for Women." *American Health,* Jan.-Feb. 1998, pp. 58–64.

wave" that will wipe people out.[9] But it needn't be a threat. Indeed, it's a formidable asset for consumer and provider alike.

There are hundreds of sites to choose from. A brief sampling is shown in Table 5.1. Health care executives and physician leaders can readily broaden their consumer education programs through the Internet. How?

- Find ways to help patients gain access to and sort through all the information out there.

- Create resource libraries, Web pages, and self-help chat rooms.

- Help patients get the information they need to be the best primary care providers that they can be.

- If your organization has an Internet Web site, be certain to have it indexed under "women's health" on all key Web browsers.

Site	Description	Address
Medscape Women's Health	This site, Medscape's electronic medical journal, has been selected for inclusion in the National Library of Medicine's Index Medicus and its online counterpart MEDLINE.	www.medscape.com
Susan G. Komen Breast Cancer Foundation	This new Web site is a comprehensive source of information on breast health and breast cancer for women concerned about their risk, as well as for current and former breast cancer patients and their families.	www.breastcancerinfo.com
Kaiser Daily Reproductive Health Report	The Kaiser Family Foundation posts this site, which features concise, up-to-date summaries of the latest news in reproductive health.	www.kff.org
National Women's Health Resource Center	This site contains information about and answers to common health questions on a variety of women's health topics, as well as links to reputable national health organization resources.	www.healthywomen.org

Table 5.1. A Sampling of Web Sites.

Now more than ever, health care organizations are desperately trying to reach out to customers and establish stronger relationships that will generate increased loyalty and repeat business. As technology such as the Internet and related media allow us to do a better job of managing information and communication, health care executives must invest the time and resources necessary to bring these new advances into the day-to-day operations of their business. Those who do will have a head start in building their brand and their customer loyalty.[10]

Providers have many options to get help needed to differentiate themselves in the market by becoming the spoke in the wheel for knowledge transfer down to the personal level. Here are three organizations that lead the chase for women's health and informed decision making:

The National Association for Women's Health (NAWH) can give you access to a community of colleagues who are experts in the field of women's health service delivery. In *Self* magazine, NAWH members' institutions accounted for over 80 percent of a list of outstanding women's centers. NAWH currently represents nearly eight hundred members across North America. The majority are women and men working in hospital-based women's health programs that support the premise that women should be informed decision makers in their own health care. Through contact with their clients, NAWH members reach one hundred thousand women each day—more than half a million each week.

NAWH can provide a health care decision maker with access to leaders who are making a women's health strategy happen in the streets. Nothing is more priceless in a competitive marketplace than real-time information about what works and what doesn't.

To get more information, contact the National Association for Women's Health at 175 W. Jackson Blvd., Suite A1711, Chicago, IL 60604. The phone number is (312) 786–1468, and the Web site address is <www.nawh.org>.

The National Women's Health Resource Center (NWHRC) can be especially helpful if your objective is to sort through the options and develop a strategy for creating a locally based clearinghouse of women's health information. Members include health professionals, women's health care centers, hospitals and health systems, corporations, government agencies, libraries, and individual consumers. NWHRC services include the National Women's Health Report;

Women's Health Fact Sheets and Learn More About . . . guides; Women's HealthInfo Searches; the NWHRC HealthWomen database; women's health information via the World Wide Web; and partnerships with organizations, associations, and corporations to enhance awareness about women's health concerns.

For more information, contact the NWHRC by mail at 5255 Loughbro Rd. N.W., Washington, DC 20016, by phone at (202) 537-4015, or by e-mail at <natlwhrc@aol.com>.

The National Women's Health Information Center (NWHIC) is an information and resource service on women's health issues designed to be accessed by the individual, whether consumer, health care professional, researcher, or woman in the military. With access through both a toll-free telephone line and on the Internet, the NWHIC acts as a federal "women's health central." Through a single point of entry, one can gain access to a vast array of women's health information available from more than a hundred federal health clearinghouses and hundreds of private sector organizations. The NWHIC is a gateway to women's health information and resources from federal health agencies, federal health clearinghouses, and World Wide Web sites related to women's health in both the public and private sectors.

The address is U.S. Public Health Service, Office on Women's Health, U.S. Department of Health and Human Services, 200 Independence Ave. S.W., Room 712E, Washington, DC 20201; phone is (800) 994-9662; Internet: <www.4woman.org>; e-mail: <4woman@asophs.dhhs.gov>.

These organizations are among an increasing host. The good news is they really help in figuring out how to best fill in the blanks of the continuum of care in a way that highlights and empowers the consumer.

SUMMARY

Due in part to gains in information technology, consumers now have considerably more data available to them. This can translate into power, making it even more important for providers to predict and meet consumers' needs, from access and convenience through sensitivity to their concerns. E-commerce creates new opportunities for customer-driven strategies. Providers who make use of the Internet to provide consumer-focused information and education will have an advantage in the years ahead.

Notes

1. Korn, P. "America's 10 Best Hospitals for Women's Care." *Self,* May 1997, p. 187.
2. Locker, R. "$4.9 Million Women's Health Center Eyed for UT." *Memphis Commercial Appeal,* Dec. 8, 1997, p. 2D.
3. Gorman, M. O. "Show Me the Coverage: Why Women Pay More for Less Health Insurance." *American Health,* Nov. 1997, p. 37.
4. "Care Providers Neglecting Birth Control Info: Study." *Nashville Tennessean,* Dec. 18, 1998, p. 10A.
5. National Center for Health Statistics. "Report of Final Mortality Statistics in 1995." *Monthly Vital Statistics Report,* 1997, *45*(11), suppl. 2.
6. Strausz, I. K. *Women's Symptoms.* New York: Dell, 1996, pp. 348–351.
7. Coombs, J. "The Role of Nutrition Screening and Intervention Programs in Managed Care." *Managed Care Quarterly,* Spring 1998, pp. 43–44.
8. "Offer Women Health Care Decision Makers High-Quality Service." *About Women & Marketing,* Oct. 1997, p. 10.
9. Fell, D. "Customer-Centered Health Care: Why Managed Care Organizations Must Capitalize on New Technology to Build Brands and Customer Loyalty." *Managed Care Quarterly,* Spring 1998, pp. 23–25.
10. Fell, "Customer-Centered Health Care."

PART TWO

Women's Health Care

Mission, Managed Care, and Market Share

T he first five chapters in this part offer specialists' points of view on areas critical to the health care marketplace. Chapter Six, by Kathleen Hanold, builds on the discussions in Chapters Three and Four about women as the drivers of public policy and market share. She emphasizes the need to reinvent health care to meet the needs of women. In Chapter Seven, Rita Menitoff asks providers to reevaluate their past approaches to competitive market dominance in order to evaluate the lessons to be learned from competition in the private sector.

The next three chapters present a variety of tools for health care: a discussion of integrated systems by Jaynelle Stichler (Chapter Eight); the social reconnaissance approach (Chapter Nine) by Michael Felix and James Burdine; and the importance of serving the underserved (Chapter Ten), written with Stacy Graham and Laura Reed. Chapter Eleven addresses ways of getting the most benefit from each marketing dollar. Together, these chapters set forth practical guidelines, from varying perspectives, on methods that are being used successfully to serve the women's health care market.

CHAPTER SIX

Success Factors for Providers of Women's Health Services

Kathleen C. Hanold

> *Kathleen C. Hanold, R.N., M.S., is vice president of women and infant services for the BJC Health System, a $1.6 billion not-for-profit integrated delivery network in St. Louis, Missouri.*

O n all fronts, women's consumer power is changing health services. What factors will define the success of a women's health strategy in the new millennium? Certainly these strategies will be different from those used in the past. Throughout the 1990s, hospitals began organizing themselves into large integrated delivery networks as a hedge (or cartel) against the tumult of managed care. Hospitals have merged into systems, acquiring everything in sight, including physicians, health plans, primary care venues, and alternative sites for care. This focus on creating mass scale and a bulk of resources has been done in an effort to drive the market, seize the competition, and survive in the chaos of managed care.

THE COMPELLING CASE FOR CHANGE

The effectiveness of greater system size is hotly debated: Is bigger better at providing the best cost, access, and service platforms, or have the corporate giants lost focus? Will the health care industry now move into an era where niche players can win?

So far, managed care seems to have focused primarily on managing cost, yet most patients report that they feel their bills are inflated. Also unfortunate is the general feeling that being cared for is increasingly lost in the hustle and bustle of complaint, diagnosis, admission, and treatment. Health systems have made valiant attempts and substantial investments to address community service, consumer satisfaction, and performance improvement. However, these efforts require resources that are in increasingly short supply. The reality is that most hospital health delivery networks have their hands full just staying in business.

To compound the complexity of the new environment, hospitals and physicians are navigating through uncharted waters of capitated and risk contracts, leading to new depths of revenue erosion and leaving a sense that very little control exists in one's practice or setting. Horror stories of managed care utilization and administrative oversight are now legion. Physicians complain of unprecedented workloads and overhead costs to comply with regulatory and health plan requirements. Health systems are learning new skills and methodologies to manage populations and covered lives. A sense of reduced control pervades the industry.

As a result of this chaos, many hospitals and health systems today find themselves awash with operating losses or reduced margins and heavily leveraged from acquisitions. Physicians find that their control, influence, and income are eroding. This, against the backdrop of declining reimbursement, means that there will probably be less capital available for health care investments. Health care is no longer a sure thing for the investment community.

FOCUSED FACTORIES AND NICHE PLAYERS COMPETE FOR MARKET SHARE

Although investors may be wary of investing in old health care models, they do understand that the market sector itself is still significant in terms of dollars. Enter the new kids on the block: niche players.[1]

Hospital systems, as new market entrants, are also facing several challenges in today's markets. For-profit niche players or investor-owned companies are beginning to change and drive competition. Regina Herzlinger, Harvard Business School professor, refers to these niche players as "focused factories," a term she borrowed from manufacturing. In her opinion, focused factories will move the health care system away from giant providers and huge managed care networks to those that have laser focus on consumer demand, convenience, and specialized care.

In *Market Driven Health Care,* Herzlinger also contends that focused-factory players concentrate on a single product line or service and aim to provide convenient one-stop shopping, unlike traditional hospitals that try to do it all with mixed results.[2] These new niche players have targeted many specialty services, including women's health, as an ideal area for investment and focus. Wall Street refers to these new niche players as "pure plays." Pure plays initially focused services that are largely ambulatory or outpatient, but now they are looking at single-specialty hospitals such as heart and women's hospitals.[3]

The traditional providers, physicians and health systems, have had mixed responses to the new market entrants. Many hospital leaders have denounced the pure-play trend as unnecessary or redundant when hospital beds remain empty in most communities today; they believe building more is wasteful. Other leaders suggest these firms are looking to provide services that cover the least sick and most insured, a phenomenon known as "cherry picking." Others discount pure plays' ability to draw the attention of patients, physicians, and health plans, believing that loyalty to the local hospital will prevail. Yet in recent market studies conducted by Women's Health Management Solutions, Inc., the traditionally held belief that a positive obstetric encounter translates to future hospital business was found to be true in only 26 percent of respondents.[4] Women shift their business based on where they can get the best care, the best service. This fact is rocking the complacent providers who thought, "If I deliver their babies, I'll have them for life."

Niche players, or focused factories, are already under scrutiny. Health plans and employers, as key customers, will be looking to evaluate the cost and quality outcomes of these new market players. Can focused women's hospitals provide services at a lower cost and also lure enough enrollee loyalty to launch a new woman-friendly service platform? Can women's medical loss ratios be better handled in a site that cares for women exclusively? Can gender-specific case management be accomplished better in a focused factory than in a megasupport hospital? These and other questions will emerge as the phenomenon of freestanding women's hospitals grows.

Not all hospital industry experts are opposed to this new trend. Some health systems may join with pure plays to bring a better product and service to market. It was not too long ago that hospitals and health systems realized that they would have to enter a competitive foray to keep their physicians in their market. Success in the future will require *reinvention* of services, not just fine-tuning in a sea of sameness. The alignment of traditional providers with the new market players could be the key to that reinvention.

REINVENTING FOR SUCCESS IN WOMEN'S HEALTH

A number of new success factors will prevail for providers of women's services in the future. Providers must recognize that consumers—especially women— are change agents and that value drives market promise. Further, businesses must be agile, develop life span relationships with women, and create partnerships with market providers.

Consumers Are Change Agents

A key trend affecting market success is the fact that consumers become agents of change and, as such, demand knowledge mastery and convenience. Regina Herzlinger refers to "consumer revolutionaries"— those individuals looking to the health care system to provide them with convenience, support to manage chronic disease, and support tools to help self-actualize or improve health status. Many of today's middle-aged female baby boomers are consumer revolutionaries, as they are the highest-earning and most educated group of women ever, as well as the fastest-growing segment of the women's market (12 percent).[5] With women making more than three-fourths of all health care decisions and representing two-thirds of the buyers and users of services, they represent a formidable market opportunity.

As an illustration, in a consumer preference study of women conducted in the St. Louis market,[6] 90 percent of women surveyed indicated that they had at least one health concern and 50 percent reported having at least one chronic condition. Seventy-four percent indicated a desire to improve their health behaviors. It became clear that significant unmet needs existed in this market. Many women desired services such as evening and weekend hours, child care, and counseling. Some reported an alarming need to frequently change physicians or insurance plans, and a lack of confidence that providers could provide current, updated women's health care. Of interest in this sample is the high out-of-pocket expenses women incurred for screening tests and alternative or complementary therapies.

The most significant finding was the degree of interest in a changed service platform: 57 percent of the women surveyed desire a different and improved service platform for health care delivery. Indeed, the desire for convenience and knowledge are clear in this illustration. It strongly suggests that preventive services must be part of a matrix of care, not just a goodwill promotional effort, for a provider of the future to be successful.

Value Proposition for the Market

Health system leaders who need to change position in the women's health market must also create a competitive advantage by coming up with a value proposition—that is, a promise to the market about how it will provide price, selection, performance, quality, convenience, and other items of value.[7] The value proposition enables a health care system to declare how it plans to compete in the market and how it will marshal the resources needed to do so.

As touched on in Chapter Four, there are three main dimensions to developing value propositions—product leadership, operational excellence, and customer intimacy:

- Product leadership means bringing the best product to market by incorporating research and development, top talent, and innovative service platforms. For the product leader in women's health, it means using gender-focused, research-based protocols and a service delivery model in which integrated providers use life span segments to identify clinical and psychosocial aspects of care delivery.

- Operational excellence requires providing a product that promotes the best total cost, maximizing efficient and effective strategies for women's health service at a price that is hard to beat. This value dimension is not usually a matter of innovation in service delivery (unless it enables efficiency) or well-developed customer relationships, but it connotes consistency. The dimension usually incorporates a key operating value, but is not usually the primary strategy to compete effectively in the women's market.

- Customer intimacy may be the most important value needed to build the best women's health care delivery system. It builds long-term relationships, identifies and meets unique needs for women, and enables the other values mentioned. Examples of this value dimension include programs that offer integrated providers in a one-stop shop with evening and weekend hours; child care, retail, and transportation services; and other features that could fulfill or exceed the unmet expectations of women.

To be successful, all three dimensions must exist. You cannot ignore efficient and effective delivery any more than you can disregard customers' unique needs or the research that enables best practice. Declaring how you want to be known in the market allows you to best position your brand of product.

Agility and Business Discipline

Health system providers face a tremendous challenge to compete effectively when pure-play providers with their focused factories enter the traditionally held clinical environment. Because pure players can focus all their efforts on a single service (unlike hospitals that juggle many), it is easier for them to get results. Improvements in customer service, minimal wait times, efficient scheduling, turnaround and throughput, multitasked staffing, and the like lead to reduced costs, convenient and satisfying consumer experiences, and attractiveness to physicians and managed care plans—to name but a few positive results. Additionally, these players can provide service platforms for physicians that improve care delivery, leaving physicians with a sense of increased control, improved earning power, and better quality of work life.

Life Span Relationships

Approximately one-third of women have their first contact with the local hospital or health system for their childbearing needs.[8] With 70 percent of the top ten surgeries occurring in women (specifically involving the reproductive system), most health systems have focused on this important but limited aspect of women's health care.[9]

But, recognizing the range of needs, the leading-edge providers of today are creating programs that consider a woman's entire life span. They are identifying clinical conditions and prevention or wellness interventions for adolescents, when lifestyle behaviors are developed that have an impact many decades later. They are considering the needs of women later in life—psychological and nutritional health, chronic conditions disproportionately affecting women, the problems of old age, and many others.

Focused factories can develop life span relationships with women under one roof, with gender-based program specialists available more readily than at hospital or health system providers because they focus on women as their only concern. This creates opportunities to market to health plan enrollees, to create evidenced-based protocols that enable best utilization, and to provide coordinated care.

SUMMARY

A number of provisos must be met in order to succeed in the sea of change that is health care today. First, providers of women's services must recognize that consumers—especially women—are change agents. They must realize that value drives market promise, and that they must be agile and develop life span relationships with women. In addition, they must create partnerships with market providers.

In today's more competitive landscape, it may be necessary to build relationships with new or different partners. When providers combine resources, they increase their ability to leverage shrinking resources or capital for investment. Ultimately, this should lead to better product and service development, lower cost, and less waste in marketing against would-be competitors. The ability to bring a new value proposition to the market should improve care, access, and service to all major stakeholders. Wouldn't it be ideal for health system providers and focused-factory pure-play providers to come to market together?

Notes

1. Peters, T. *Circle of Innovation.* New York: Knopf, 1997, pp. 399–425.
2. Herzlinger, R. *Market Driven Health Care: Who Wins, Who Loses in the Transformation of America's Largest Service Industry.* Reading, Mass.: Perseus Books, 1997, pp. 163–201.
3. Health Care Advisory Board. *Partnership at Risk: The Precarious State of Specialist/Health System Relations.* Washington, D.C.: Health Care Advisory Board, 1988.

4. "Women's Health Management Solutions." Unpublished research findings. BJC Health System, 1998.

5. "FY 1996 Population Demographics." Unpublished research findings. BJC Health System, 1997.

6. "Women's Health Management Solutions."

7. Treacy, M., and Wiersema, F. *The Discipline of Market Leaders.* Reading, Mass.: Addison-Wesley, 1995, pp. 31–45.

8. National Center for Health Statistics. *Facts About Women.* Washington, D.C.: National Center for Health Statistics, 1994.

9. Wilmoth, M., and Malone, A. *The New Women's Movement: Women's Healthcare.* Smith Barney Research, 1997.

CHAPTER SEVEN

Private Sectors and the Women's Health Market

Rita J. Menitoff

> *Rita J. Menitoff is founder and president of Women's Health Management Solutions, LLC, in New York City. She was formerly senior consultant and women's health practice leader for Computer Science Corporation– American Practice Management, Inc.*

New investor-owned organizations are changing the rules in the women's health care arena by challenging traditional service providers to rethink their strategies. As the health care market evolves toward greater consolidation and integration of entrenched hospital systems, new players are leap-frogging market entry barriers. Private sector entrepreneurs are attracting consumers, insurers, and clinicians. Investor-owned systems are accelerating competition by setting new standards in pricing, cost reduction, physician gain sharing, and medical innovation. Is this competition and the entry of the private sector good for women's health? Will this serious competitive environment result in more women receiving medically appropriate health care? In considering these questions, we discuss the market for women's health, how health care now fails women, private sector opportunities, and new models.

WOMEN'S HEALTH IS A HUGE MARKET

The point cannot be overemphasized: Women rule in the health care market. They are, as Tom Peters asserts, economic opportunity number one.[1] They spend $121 billion on health care, only $40.7 billion of which goes toward reproductive services.[2] Why boomer women—with their mothers and daughters—rule the health care market can be explained by six trends:

- *Policymaking:* The majority of women voted for Clinton.
- *Spending:* Women account for 60 percent of the total medical bill for the United States.[3]
- *Knowledge:* 46 percent of all Internet users are women.[4]
- *Demographics:* Nearly 50 percent of the labor force will be female by the year 2006, and birth rates are declining.[5]
- *Aging:* 53 million women will reach menopause in the next ten years, and more than half of them see it as a new beginning.[6]
- *Utilization:* Women account for 60 percent of all doctor's visits.[7]

Women are about half of the population, but over two-thirds of the buyers and users of health care services (over $500 billion annually).[8] They consume 66 percent of the health care dollar; make 75 percent of health care decisions; generate 56 percent of all ambulatory surgeries; and represent 75 percent of nursing home patients.[9] Women over forty in America are the highest-earning group of women ever. Now and for the next twenty years they will have more spending power than any other generation. When it comes to health care, women are demanding less invasive procedures, alternative and complementary therapies, lifestyle convenience, credible gender-specific information, inclusion in care decisions, and more practitioner face time.

HEALTH CARE FAILS WOMEN

The existing system is not working for women, and the voices calling for change are escalating. Study after study documents their dissatisfaction with both the financing and delivery of health care. A growing body of evidence confirms that this lack of confidence in conventional medical practice and existing system configurations is well founded; past failures to appreciate sex differences in health, disease, diagnosis, and treatment, and in the design of delivery systems, medications, or medical devices have clearly led to deficits or gaps in health care for women.

Recent findings from gender-based medical research have left physicians clinically stranded as a growing gap emerges between important new findings from clinical trials and the reeducation of physicians who typically provide care. This new challenge arises as the long-standing inattention to the study of health problems experienced by women and a lack of their fair share of scientific resources is being addressed. In 1990 the Office of Research in Women's Health committed $625 million to the Women's Health Initiative, and in 1992 the FDA repealed its exclusion of women from clinical trials. The resulting flood of research conclusions renders historic approaches to diagnosis and treatment of women obsolete. Examples abound: from cardiovascular disease and stroke to depression and bipolar disorders—medications and test results have a different impact on women than on men. A transfer of research findings from academic medicine to community practice is a slow process involving the teaching and retooling of physicians and other practitioners.

Managed care also contributes to gaps in care. Women's health has become a managed care nemesis: coverage issues have become political lightning rods distracting management attention and resources from outcomes research and benchmarking efforts. Managed care is under siege. It needs to attract women as enrollees and at the same time reduce their utilization (a 75 percent higher medical loss ratio for women).[10] Issues such as "drive-through" deliveries and mastectomies, breast implants, pap smears, Viagra versus contraception, cosmetic surgery, and genetic screening—all gender-related considerations—are the most hotly debated issues in health care today.

Women find it difficult to rely on their regular physician of the past who may not be up to date in gender-based medical advances and who may not be in the network of their managed care plan. This dissatisfaction may be reflected in the nearly 50 percent of women who have turned to alternative therapies to supplement their traditional health care.[11] The problem is compounded by the fact that the boundaries between specialty and primary care clinicians serving women are disintegrating as care is integrating. Most plans designate an internist or family practitioner as gatekeeper but allow a primary care visit to an OB/GYN, perpetuating fragmented care. Many women (70 percent of reproductive-age women in one major Midwest market)[12] look to women's health centers to get the health care they want. Although many of these centers focus only on women, they remain inherently fragmented. The majority are reproductive only; others are multi-specialty but not team-based, and offer many nonreimbursable preventive screening and diagnostic services.

Another potential source of comprehensive integrated health care for women—the integrated delivery system—is burdened by the same general issues that limit their effectiveness. Health services scholar Steven Shortell discovered in his multihospital study in 1996 that the relationship between overall integration and the systems' hospital performance was not impressive.[13] Without integration at the point of care, health care systems will continue to fail women. Women, in particular, are experiencing the breakdown of these delivery and financing systems without a suitable replacement. What women are getting is not what they want, either for themselves or for their families.

PRIVATE SECTOR OPPORTUNITIES

Will women's health follow the same private sector trends as general health care? Fertility centers, birthing centers, OB/GYN group practices, cosmetic surgery centers, and alternative medicine centers are showing up as niche market players across the nation. These niche players—or "focused factories," as they are sometimes called (see Chapter Six)—enable the high volume necessary for technical competency and economies of scale. In women's health, they are characterized by convenient one-stop shopping and out-of-pocket purchasing opportunities that represent approximately $40 billion in nonmedical remedies in women's health. Venture capitalists have already invested 10 percent of the health care dollar in women's health, transferring from biotechnology to physician practice management (PPMs) because of their faster return.[14] These women's health ventures tend to follow general trends in the health care sector, such as growth in advertising to attract women patients. Wall Street knows that the demographics alone should add up to profit. There is the same risk of small companies specializing in high-tech breakthroughs in women's health. There are even a few security analysts specializing in the sector. These analysts believe that many of the stocks did not meet investor expectations in the bull market because they went public prematurely.[15] Less-than-exciting results can be explained by FDA approval lags, the slow process of replacing community practice, and the inexperience in management and public relations of women's health entrepreneurs. As with other health care growth areas, the new direction of acquisitions by big pharmaceutical and medical device companies is proving more interesting to investors.

In part, the success of the private sector is due to the weak competitive response of the traditional nonprofit health care institutions. Historical loyalties are breaking down. As mentioned in an earlier chapter, only 26 percent of women choose the hospital in which they gave birth for subsequent non-maternity-related admissions. Fifty-six percent of women change their primary care physicians at least once every five years, and 10 percent change three or more times during that period.[16] Consumers are turning to the private sector to meet their needs. The proliferation of calcium supplements, health fitness clubs, at-home exercise equipment, and easy-to-prepare frozen meals are a rapid response to some of the preventive services and convenience products women are demanding.

Health care organizations tend to view the need for gender-based medical approaches as merely a customer service issue rather than a reorientation in medical practice. The same institutions continue to squabble over control of turf in reduction of excess capacity. Furthermore, the traditional hospital systems cannot compete with powerful Internet and intranet technology to integrate care process information and reach the consumer with health information. The private sector can move much more quickly to identify and mobilize technology and professionals to employ new gender-specific medical approaches without distraction of multiple missions, tenured staff, outdated systems, and, more importantly, lack of incentive to change. Hospital systems need dramatically more effective initiatives to secure their women's health market share. Rather than focusing on billing and collections, bonuses, advertising existing services, and painting the walls pink, they need to transform their existing resources into a women-centered model—comprehensive, integrated, convenient, and up-to-date.

NEW MODELS

What then is the best strategy to deliver the highest-quality medical care at the most reasonable cost? New models of women's health partnerships that involve all stakeholder groups are needed to truly improve women's health. Pure-play entrepreneurial ventures are focused and innovative but financially fragile and limited in scope. The enormous megahealth system institutions are struggling to provide value from their size. Both sectors—public and private—together can provide the development, deployment, and distribution of women's health products and services in complementary relationships.

The product development cycle can be a good illustration of the interdependence of the two sectors in advancing women's health services. Consider what happens when a pharmaceutical company and an academic teaching and research center develop a new technology in women's health. Together, they recruit patients, conduct clinical trials, and train providers. The pharmaceutical company funds the development of protocols and outcome analysis in the provider institution. Reimbursement mechanisms are negotiated with managed care which then establishes the new technology as standard community practice. In this scenario, the public and private sectors have collaborated to produce and deliver better health care to women; all stakeholders are included.

A growing number of women's health partnership opportunities have created new standards of care; one prominent example is Cytyc Company's Thinprep for cervical cancer screening. Universal managed care coverage is pending; in the meantime, women are already paying out-of-pocket for a more accurate result. Another case is Columbia Labs, which by attracting American Home Products to its Columbia University team has seen sales of its natural progesterone applicator grow fivefold to $6 million.[17] This public-private partnership overcame a market entry barrier of scale. The most dramatic example in advancing gender-specific medicine is the collaboration between Columbia University and four other academic and teaching institutions to establish GenCite—the first comprehensive electronic database in gender-based research.[18]

As managed care continues to look for cost-effective strategies in women's health, providers and provider systems are encouraged to develop evidence that the approaches they are using drive down costs without harming health status. Clinical research is focused on evidence-based medicine. These investigations typically involve hundreds of physicians, statisticians, information technology, data warehouses, and large patient populations to be studied. These studies are being funded by companies such as Genentech, Ciba-Geigy, Hoffman La Roche, and Glaxo in partnership with integrated delivery systems and managed care. In a move toward less invasive gynecologic surgery, medical equipment manufacturers such as US Surgical are now funding promising new procedures using microscopic and laser surgery, thus making possible smaller incisions, quicker surgeries, less opportunity for infection, and shorter hospital stays.

These new medical technologies are shifting the setting and approach of many inpatient women's health services, including high-risk pregnancy and gynecologic surgery as well as assisted reproductive technology, cosmetic surgery, and urogynecology. To compete in the women's health marketplace, delivery systems must invest in the technologies of the twenty-first century: core needle biopsy, minimally invasive gynecologic surgery, prenatal home monitoring, genetic testing, genome science, and high-dose chemotherapy with stem cell support. These new procedures will create a demand in all markets by patients and physicians that managed care will treat as community practice.

Delivery systems are creating whole new models of care delivery: mind-body primary care; low-intensity model hospitals (birthing centers); a critical mass of high-end services, such as infertility, consolidated in a few sites; and bringing services closer to the consumer (telemetry).

Niches are developing in the women's health market around conditions of high prevalence or concern to women. These specialty niches concentrate resources and position specialists and marketing in areas such as urogynecology and incontinence programs, high-risk pregnancies, gynecologic oncology (where sizable profit margins draw top physicians), supplier investments, research, and teaching opportunities.

Hospital systems use their existing platforms in clinical pathways, databases, and managed care relationships to compete in the women's health market. However, these new models are risky. They require focused management, a scale large enough to concentrate volume in a customer segment, and low-cost operation. Most importantly, to win in women's health product lines, physicians must be your partners. Physicians need to see professional and secure futures for themselves in the health care system of the future.

Physicians who are involved in women's health are in a state of professional turmoil. Male OB/GYNs especially may be in oversupply in most markets, as many women prefer female physicians. Female internists and family practitioners are attracting women for primary care but may not have the training necessary for reproductive care. Increasingly, physicians resent being employees and are much more attracted to ownership and investment in the success of the enterprise, with the emphasis being on demonstration of effectiveness. They are also attracted to organizations that can provide data and information at the point of service and gender-based protocols. On a professional level, many aspire to be leaders of women's health service product lines and select those opportunities that provide income maximization over income guarantees.

One option, to bring together the advances in clinical research, medical technology, and delivery system reform and maximize the impact of women's health initiatives, is cross-industry partnership. To succeed, all partners—physicians, hospitals, managed care, and business investors—must clearly define their relationship. Partnering can occur anywhere on a continuum from a loose traditional partnership to a tight alliance and strategic partnership. When the roles of these partners are unclear, the partnerships create tentative involvement at best and aggressive behaviors at worst, leading to disastrous results for the enterprise. Another factor in sustaining these new models is building consumer trust in public-private collaborations. A survey commissioned by the Kaiser Family Foundation and Harvard found that 65 percent of the population believes that incentives threaten the quality of care.[19] Consumer representation on the boards of these enterprises is a necessity. Hospital advertising is a good example of the manifestation of the ethical challenges in women's health. Consider, for example, the fact that in 1984, $104 million was spent in hospital advertising and, by 1996, $1.28 billion.[20] When does a woman's survival story of breast cancer treatment become misleading? Are the dollars allocated to advertising and marketing women's product lines better spent on research or providing care to the underserved?

Ultimately, the partners must create a women's health enterprise that will lead the market in three areas: operational excellence, customer lifestyle intimacy, and gender medicine. Sample value propositions for each of these follow:

- *Operational excellence across the continuum.* The full continuum of care is available to women in a one-stop health center, a twenty-four-hour-a-day, seven-days-a-week call line, same-day urgent care near the worksite, and day care within the facility. Each woman has one medical record so her OB/GYN, internist, and specialist can coordinate care.

- *Customer lifestyle intimacy.* All practitioners understand and are responsive to needs for gender information, convenient access, compassion, respect, and confidentiality. A woman is treated as a total person, not a collection of body parts. All health concerns—those of mind and body—are taken seriously. Personal health risks are analyzed and follow-up on compliance is provided.

- *Leadership in gender medicine.* The highest-quality women's health specialist and women-specific medical research programs and advance technologies are focused in important medical conditions of adolescent, reproductive, mid-life, and senior women. Evidence-based research provides insurance companies with the port for benefit coverage and preferred provider status.

The members of the partnership must jointly decide the structure and future of the venture. They must decide who will provide the right combination of competencies to reach clinical and financial goals. Each member of the partnership brings different capabilities that are distinctive, complementary, or fall short of the competitive level needed in their market. The partnership must decide if the resources should be owned or contracted, developed internally, or outsourced. As long as each is focused on what it does best and shares in the success of the others, the partnership has a good prognosis. Building the capacity to deliver value in operational excellence, customer lifestyle intimacy, and gender medicine leadership will be the challenge. Ultimately, each partner must decide whether the collective relationship will optimize its vision or if redesigning its own women's health program will be the better approach.

SUMMARY

It is clear today that irreversible gains in women's health and gender medicine will create new opportunities for public-private collaborations. Many issues revolving around conflict between mission and stockholder value will challenge the survival of these relationships.

Four propositions support increasing integration of private sector players in the women's health market:

- Women's health is the biggest health care market in history now and in the foreseeable future. The economic outlook is good.

• The classic health care delivery system fails miserably to serve women. This creates unmet demand.

• The private sector is attracted to the market size opportunity and to the chaos and vulnerability of the entrenched players, institutions, and physicians.

• New models are inevitable yet risky; partnership may mitigate the risks.

Is the private sector a long-term player in women's health? Will innovative new technologies and models replace cumbersome bureaucracies of the public sector? These are questions that providers must consider, and consider carefully, to succeed in the competitive women's health care market.

Notes

1. Peters, T. *The Circle of Innovation.* New York: Knopf, 1997, p. 410.
2. Women's Research and Education Institute. *Women's Health Insurance Costs and Experiences.* Washington, D.C.: Women's Research and Education Institute, 1994.
3. Women's Research and Education Institute, *Women's Health Insurance Costs and Experiences.*
4. CyberStats. [http://www.mediamark.com/pages/freedata.htm]. 1998.
5. U.S. Bureau of the Census. *Statistical Abstract of the United States, 1998.* Washington, D.C.: U.S. Government Printing Office, 1998, p. 403.
6. Kaufert, P., and others. "Women and Menopause: Beliefs, Attitudes and Behaviors—The NAMS 1997 Menopause Survey." *Menopause,* 1998, 5(4), 197–202.
7. Lipkind, K. L. "National Hospital Ambulatory Medical Care Survey: 1993 Outpatient Department Summary." Advance data from *Vital Statistics,* no. 276, Hyattsville, Md., 1996.
8. Smith Barney Research. *The New Women's Movement: Women's Health Insurance Costs and Experiences.* Washington, D.C.: Smith Barney Research, 1994.
9. Katz, P. *The Feminist Dollar: The Wise Woman's Buying Guide.* New York: Plenum, 1997; Peters, *Circle of Innovation,* p. 398; U.S. National Center for Health Statistics, Advance Data, no. 300, Aug. 12, 1998; U.S. National Center for Health Statistics, Advance Data, no. 289, July 2, 1997.

10. WHMS client experiences.
11. Eisenberg, D. "Trends in Alternative Medicine Use in the United States, 1990–1997." *Journal of the American Medical Association,* 1998, *280,* 1569–1575.
12. WHMS client experiences.
13. Shortell, S. "KPMG Multi-Hospital Study," 1996.
14. Price Waterhouse Venture Capital Study, 1997.
15. Eaton, L. "Researchers Finding New Wariness on Wall Street." *New York Times,* June 21, 1998, p. WH8.
16. WHMS market research.
17. Marcial, G. "Feeling a Rush at Columbia Labs." *Business Week,* Apr. 1, 1996, p. 80.
18. Baumgardner, J. "Science + Corporate Bucks = Health Revolution?" *Ms.,* May-June 1998, pp. 34–36.
19. "Kaiser/Harvard University Survey of Americans' Views on the Consumer Protection Debate." 1998.
20. Kornblut, A. "As Hospitals Step Up Ads, Issues of Cost, Ethics Arise." *Boston Globe,* Aug. 25, 1998, p. 25.

CHAPTER EIGHT

Integrated Systems of Care for Women's Health

Jaynelle F. Stichler

> *Jaynelle F. Stichler, D.N.S., is a principal in charge of the Healthcare Division at the Stichler Group, Inc., in San Diego. Her work is recognized throughout the nation and internationally in Australia, Mexico, Korea, Thailand, and Malaysia.*

The concept of system integration is relatively new to the health care industry. Before the late 1980s, there were very few health care systems, and most of these were large national chains that owned several hospitals within one state or across several states. Now, to improve their negotiating positions with managed care and prospective payment systems for health care reimbursement, many hospitals have merged, associated, affiliated, or otherwise joined to develop strong systems that are vertically integrated with physicians and payors and horizontally integrated across various entities within the system.

The development of service lines or product line management facilitated the bundling of similar services into strategic business units to promote marketing, to enhance operational efficiencies, and to advance quality improvement and research initiatives. The women's service line is one example of bundled services that are often seen in health care systems. Although the service line can continue separately as maternity, gynecology, infertility, breast surgery, and other related services for women, the benefits of combining all the services into a system of care for women are readily apparent. The purpose of this chapter is to explore the benefits and barriers to developing integrated systems of care for women's health and to identify strategies that can facilitate the integration process.

DEFINING THE WOMEN'S HEALTH SERVICE LINE

The first step to integrating the women's service line is to define the service line specifically. Women's health is defined differently in each organization. To some it equates to the maternity service line and often includes infant services (normal newborn and neonatal intensive care) as well. The most comprehensive definition includes those conditions that exist in women only, occur with women more frequently, or affect women differently. Generally, this definition leads to the inclusion of the following programs and services for the women's service line: fertility services, perinatal care, gynecology (GYN) care, urogynecology, gyn-oncology, and breast health services.

When the service line is expanded to include women's health, services such as health education, support services, integrative therapies, lifestyle and fitness screening, and behavioral health will likely be included. The diagnostic related groups (DRGs) that are often included in the women's service line are shown in Table 8.1. This service line includes not only inpatient diagnoses but outpatient visits for screening, education, and interventions.

It is important to define this service line clearly because of its overlap with other service lines. Although most organizations focus on reproduction as the anchor tenant for the women's service line, few women actually experience morbidity or mortality with childbirth or gynecological events requiring hospitalization or outpatient visits. The real insults to women's health are often quite separate from reproduction.

When one considers the significant threats to the health and wellbeing of women, reproductive issues pale in comparison to heart disease, cancer, and other potential problems. For example, osteoporosis affects nearly twenty-four million American women annually and

Table 8.1.   Diagnostic Related Groups (DRGs)
for Women's Health Services.

DRG	Category	Description
Women's Cancer (Breast and Gynecology)		
257	Surgery	Total Mastectomy for Malignancy w/Complication
258	Surgery	Total Mastectomy for Malignancy w/o Complication
259	Surgery	Subtotal Mastectomy for Malignancy w/Complication
260	Surgery	Subtotal Mastectomy for Malignancy w/o Complication
352	Surgery	Pelvic Evisceration, Radical Hysterectomy and Radical Vulvectomy
354	Surgery	Uterine, Adnexa Procedure for Nonovarian/Adnexal Malignancy w/cc
355	Surgery	Uterine, Adnexa Procedure for Nonovarian/Adnexal Malignancy w/o cc
357	Surgery	Uterine and Adnexa Procedures for Ovarian or Adnexal Malignancy
358	Surgery	Uterine and Adnexa Procedures for Nonmalignancy w/cc
359	Surgery	Uterine and Adnexa Procedures for Nonmalignancy w/o cc
Gynecology		
356	Surgery	Female Reproductive System Reconstructive Procedures
360	Surgery	Vagina, Cervix and Vulva Procedures
361	Surgery	Laparoscopy and Incisional Tubal Interruption
362	Surgery	Endoscopic Tubal Interruption
364	Surgery	D&C Conization Except for Malignancy
365	Surgery	Other Female Reproductive System O.R. Procedures
368	Medical	Infections, Female Reproductive System
369	Medical	Menstual and Other Female Reproductive System Disorders
Nonmalignant Breast Disorders		
261	Surgery	Breast Procedure for Nonmalignant Except Biopsy and Local Excision
262	Surgery	Breast Biopsy and Local Excision for Nonmalignancy
276	Medical	Nonmalignant Breast Disorders
Women's Genitourinary		
308[a]	Surgery	Minor Bladder Procedures w/cc
309[a]	Surgery	Minor Bladder Procedures w/o cc
Obstetrical and Related		
370	Surgery	Cesarean Section w/cc
371	Surgery	Cesarean Section w/o cc
374	Surgery	Vaginal Delivery w/Sterilization and/or D&C
375	Surgery	Vaginal Delivery w/O.R. Proc Except Sterile and/or D&O
377	Surgery	Postpartum and Postabortion Diagnoses w/O.R. Procedure
381	Surgery	Abortion w/D&C Aspiration Curettage or Hysterotomy
372	Medical	Vaginal Delivery w/Complicating Dx
373	Medical	Vaginal Delivery w/o Complicating Dx

DRG	Category	Description
376	Medical	Postpartum and Postabortion Dx w/o O.R. Procedure
378	Medical	Ectopic Pregnancy
379	Medical	Threatened Abortion
380	Medical	Abortion w/o D&C
383	Medical	Other Antepartum Dx w/Medical Complications
384	Medical	Other Antepartum Diagnoses w/o Medical Complications

Normal Newborns

391	Medical	Normal Newborns
388	Medical	Premature w/o Major Problems

Neonates and Problems at Birth

385	Medical	Neonates Died or Transferred to Another Acute Care Facility
386	Medical	Extreme Immaturity or Respiratory Distress Syndrom, Neonate
387	Medical	Prematurity w/Major Problems
389	Medical	Full-Term Neonate w/Major Problems
390	Medical	Neonate w/Other Significant Problems

[a]Data runs are currently under way to determine if this DRG should be included or excluded.

results in three hundred thousand hip fractures annually and subsequent death in older women. Considering that nearly one in four women suffer from depressive disorders after the age of forty, the behavioral health service line becomes an important partner with women's health as well.[1] The senior service line also has significant overlap, as the majority of seniors are women. But without doubt, heart disease and cancer rank right at the top.

Women and Heart Disease

According to the American Heart Association, heart and cardiovascular disease is the number one killer of American women.[2] Of the approximately 485,000 heart attack deaths each year, nearly half occur in women. Another 87,000 die each year from strokes. It is now known that the woman's risk for cardiovascular disease increases after the onset of menopause. Does this make heart disease an issue to be considered in the women's health service line? Absolutely! Cardiac care and interventional therapies need to be in the cardiac service line, because the concentration of expertise and shared knowledge about the disease process and the interventions exist there. Clearly there is an overlap between the two service lines, and the greatest overlap exists between the prevention of heart disease and women's health. When health education programs are provided for the community labeled as "Preventing Heart Disease," few women attend. Those that do attend often do so to gather information to prevent heart disease for their husbands or partners. When the program is titled "Women and Heart Disease" or "Estrogen Use and Its Effect on Heart Disease in Women," however, there likely will be standing room only. Women are innately tuned in to health education and care that is prepared specifically for them or information on specific symptoms that they or a friend or loved one is experiencing.

Women and Cancer

Cancer services are very similar to cardiac services in their overlap with the women's service line. The prevention, early detection, and intervention of cancer are significant; screening and early detection of breast cancer with mammography is an "anchor tenant" in the women's service line. Feedback from women obtained in focus groups indicates that most women prefer to go to a women's health center or a stand-alone breast center for their annual mammography rather than going to a breast center that is a part of a cancer center. However, if a suspicious area is detected, most women want to go to the best cancer center possible for diagnosis and intervention.

Breast cancer is a significant concern to women, and nearly forty-four thousand of them die annually from the disease. Nearly fifty-three thousand women die annually from lung cancer. Health education targeted specifically to women about the dangers and prevention of lung cancer and the early detection of breast cancer should be developed jointly between the women's and cancer service lines.

Services for cancers that are specific to women or that occur more frequently in women can be a part of both service lines. Because the expertise and body of knowledge for cancer care exists in the cancer service line, most conditions requiring radical surgical intervention and long-term chemotherapy or radiation therapy are cared for in the cancer service line. More simplistic cases of gynecology/oncology and some surgical cases of noncomplicated breast disease can be included in the women's service line. The overlap between the two service lines is seen more clearly in the prevention and early detection of cancer.

The importance of collaborative planning and program development among systemwide service lines is readily apparent. Not only does each service line need to be integrated across the system, but all the service lines within the system also need to be integrated among them. One advantage to integration within the service line or collaboratively with other services is that it allows the sharing of resources and expertise and expands the knowledge and sensitivity to women's health among all providers. When service lines begin to work together collaboratively or when hospitals work together within the same service line, the groups begin to know, trust, and value each other more. True integration will only occur as a result of collaborative effort built on a platform of trust, sharing, and balance of power.

Figure 8.1 displays the universe of programs and services that can be considered within the women's health service line. The degree to which all or part of the programs exist within women's services or in other service lines is not important, so long as the programs are available and packaged in a manner that will attract women.

USING ORGANIZATIONAL STRUCTURE TO ENHANCE INTEGRATION EFFORTS

There are as many different organizational designs of integrated health care systems as there are organizations. When developing an organizational structure to facilitate clinical system integration, the following must be considered:

- The geographical proximity of the respective hospitals or entities within the system
- The level of integration of management decision support systems such as finance, management information systems, and human resources
- The degree to which corporate support systems such as planning and marketing, purchasing, and executive decision making are integrated
- The expectation and rewards that have been communicated by top management in support of integration

The design of the organization is critical and should be carefully considered, because it provides the framework on which all systems and integrative efforts will be developed. The organizational structure can either enhance or inhibit the integration and effect the organization's ability to achieve stated goals. Hospitals are traditionally complex organizations that have been organized around specific clinical

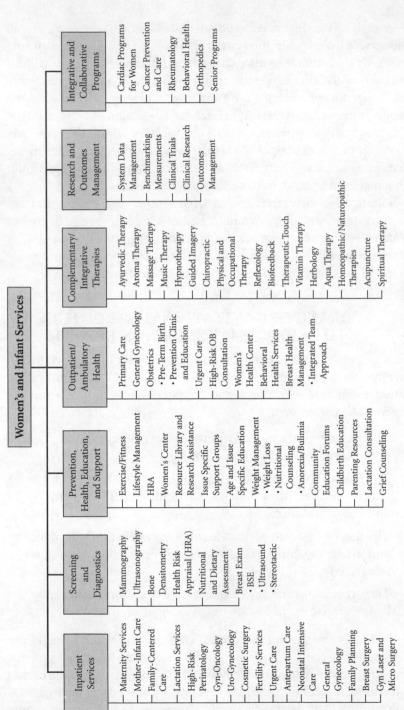

Figure 8.1. Universe of Programs and Services.

specialties or support services; ownership is clear in specific clinical or support territories. When systemwide needs are superimposed on an already rigid organizational structure, integration efforts become even more difficult.

The first step in the design of the new organization is to redefine service line and support service boundaries. The span of control may need to extend beyond the boundaries of one hospital into several others within the system. It may also be necessary to develop a structure that crosses traditional organizational departments and boundaries. This is particularly true in a system that has hospitals and other health care entities within close proximity. We will review three different organizational structures—matrix, parallel, and single point of direction—that have been implemented in some health care systems across the nation to facilitate the integration of women's health services and other service lines.

Matrix Structures

As with most matrix structures, individuals may report to several people. For example, one health care system in the Midwest uses a matrix system for organizing its women's service line. A regional director for women's health services reports to a regional vice president for clinical services, who has responsibility for all clinical service lines. Both individuals have responsibilities for service-line direction in three hospitals in an urban setting. In this system, one hospital is a tertiary hospital in the inner city; a second is a tertiary hospital for cardiac and cancer care but does not provide tertiary-level care for women's services; and a third provides community-level services, including a low-volume maternal-newborn program. All hospitals are located within ten miles of each other.

The regional director for women's health services is responsible for the strategic planning, program development, and coordination of integration efforts for that service line, including inpatient clinical services, education and support services, and research and quality initiatives. The position is also responsible for directing business development in collaboration with the planning and marketing department. Outpatient services for women's health are planned and coordinated with the regional director for ambulatory services.

In addition to the strategic duties described, the regional director for women's health has clinical managers for each specific clinical service, such as the family birthing centers, maternal-newborn care, or gynecology services at each hospital. For the operational side of clinical care management, the regional director reports directly to the chief operating officer at each hospital. In this role, the director is responsible for the budget management, staffing, and quality initiatives for each hospital. In this matrix model (see Figure 8.2), the director is responsible for strategic systemwide functions and local entity-based operations, and reports directly to several individuals in the organization.

There are several advantages to this matrix model of management for the integration of women's health and other service lines. For one, strategic planning and program development is initiated and coordinated from a single source at the system level. This eliminates much of the political positioning that occurs when multiple entity leaders come together at the system level to plan and coordinate programs. Although system planning occurs at the corporate level, the specific needs of each entity are addressed because the director is also responsible at each entity for the operational success of the service line at the local level.

The model is also integrated across functions, because the regional manager must collaborate closely with the planning and marketing department, the physician development department, and other clinical service line regional directors to be successful in the role. The "forced" interdependence fosters collaborative and integrative efforts.

Parallel Structure Models

There are several variations to the parallel structure model. In one, two system directors for the women's health or other service lines

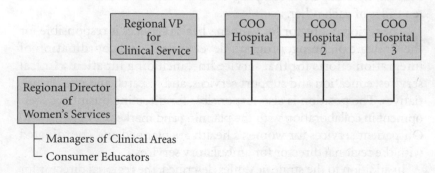

Figure 8.2. Matrix Model of Organizational Design.

share responsibility and accountability for the service line. This model is illustrated in Figure 8.3.

Both directors have corporate and systemwide responsibilities, but each focuses on a specific part of the role. The system director for clinical operations for women's services has several clinical managers from each system entity reporting to the person in this role. Collectively, they are responsible for budget management, staffing, and quality initiatives including clinical policies and procedures, interprofessional relationships, and the like. The system director for women's services is responsible for the strategic planning, program development, business development, and integration of clinical services and support services for all entities. In this role, the system director does not have direct reports but must work collaboratively with the corporate planning and marketing department, physician groups, the corporate finance and contracts department for service pricing and contract negotiations, and other service line directors for coordination of services specifically targeted to women.

The advantages of this model include specific emphasis on two important aspects of the job, clinical operations and strategic planning, by two individuals focused on each area. It is rare to find one individual who has the skill set necessary for the combined role of planning and operations. For large systems with multiple entities or large volume women's health departments, the division of the role creates a more realistic span of control and responsibility.

Problems can develop with the parallel model if the two system directors are not able to work together. Any sense of divisiveness or

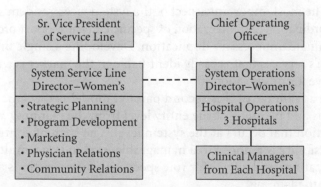

Figure 8.3.   Parallel Shared Responsibility Administrative Structure.

difference in direction for the service line will present conflict and confusion at all levels within the organization. The directors must also be clear on the scope and boundaries of their roles. As an example, if a physician were concerned about a specific clinical issue, it would not be wise for the system director for strategic planning to become involved in the investigation and resolution of the problem unless the issue has a global perspective and strategic implications. Even then, the resolution must involve the system director for operations who is responsible for the operational aspects at the clinical level.

In a second parallel model, illustrated in Figure 8.4, each entity has a clinical director of women's services who has line responsibilities and is responsible for operations including budget management, staffing, and quality initiatives. In addition, the clinical directors are responsible for strategic planning and program development for their entity. The clinical directors report directly to the chief operating officer or chief nursing officer at each entity, but have a collaborative relationship with the system vice president for women's services.

The system vice president for the women's service line is responsible for strategic planning, program development, operational assessment, business development, and community outreach activities for the service line. In some organizations this person is also responsible for quality and research initiatives and for marketing and promotional activities including fundraising. These last few roles are performed in collaboration with the corporate planning and marketing departments and the corporate and entity-specific foundations that are ultimately responsible for fundraising. The position usually does not have line responsibility and often reports to a senior executive (senior vice president) responsible for the system planning and initiatives for all service lines. The most important aspect of the system vice president's role is the coordination and integration of specific clinical support programs to eliminate unnecessary duplication. Developing a single brand of women's services that is easily identifiable in the market is a critical initiative for this position.

The advantage of this second parallel model is the split in operations and planning at the entity level from the planning and coordination that occurs at the system level. The span of control and responsibility is reduced to a manageable level in large, multientity organizations and allows for role specificity for operations as contrasted to planning.

Major political problems are often seen in this organizational model as the clinical directors compete to protect their entity's specific

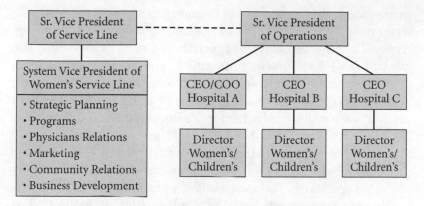

Figure 8.4.   Parallel Service Line Structure.

interests and initiatives over those of the system. Because the clinical directors report up through the hierarchy of their entity, and the system director or vice president reports up through a different reporting structure, there are many opportunities for power plays, political positioning, and sabotage. The system vice president for women's services, being a staff position, relies on power by expertise and persuasion. The clinical director has vested power in the position to make changes to promote the entity's interests, even at the expense of other system players.

Although is it expected that clinical directors and the system vice president will work collaboratively, in many organizations the latter is hindered because of the battle for control of the service line. Clearly, a lot of energy is expended with this model on positioning, power brokering, persuading, and protecting rather than on strategies to neutralize external competition.

Competition and conflict can also occur at top executive levels of the organization in this model as each executive sees problems from their directors' perspective rather than from a system perspective. At times it would seem that the system and its members are in direct competition in this model.

Single Point of Direction Model

There are several variations of single point of direction models, but the one most frequently seen is similar to the second parallel model just described. The major point of distinction is in the reporting structure.

In this model, all clinical directors or managers report to the system director or vice president for the service line, who is responsible for operations, strategic planning, program development, quality initiatives, research, fund development, community outreach, and integration of clinical programs in collaboration with other management support departments (corporate planning and marketing, foundation, clinical research, and quality) and other service line directors. Another major difference in this model is that the clinical directors do not report up through the hierarchy of the entity or hospital. Instead, each reports to the system vice president (VP), who is also accountable for the integrity of clinical operations. This model is illustrated in Figure 8.5.

The system VP reports operational information to the entity chief executive or chief operational officer and planning and integration information to the system's senior executive responsible for service line integration.

This model eliminates most of the political positioning seen in the second parallel model. It provides a single point of focus for service line definition, planning, program development, and operations for the entire system. This model truly fosters clinical integration because all planning is done from the system level even for the specific needs of each entity that must be sensitive and responsive at the local community level. In essence, the system becomes responsible for the success of each entity as well as the system as a whole. The philosophy underpinning this model is that if one part suffers, the whole system will suffer.

In large, geographically dispersed systems, this model may have an unreasonable span of control and responsibility. If there are great distances between the entities, the system VP may frequently be unavailable to the clinical director, who will ultimately use the usual upward communication through the entity rather than through the system service line structure. Doing so may create conflict among the executive leadership at both levels.

WOMEN'S SERVICE LINE DIRECTORS' ROLES

The women's health service line vice president (director) should not be aligned with any one entity or to an inpatient setting. Ensuring a nonentity bias in the strategic planning and coordination of programs is critical for an integrated service line. A nonaligned position can facilitate a balanced direction for the service line, including the indi-

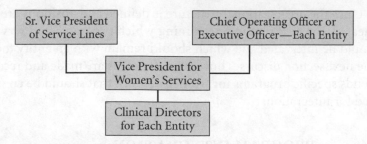

Figure 8.5.   System Model for Single Point of Direction.

vidual and collective needs of inpatient and outpatient settings for women's health.

The skills of the service line director should include knowledge of women's health and specific skill and expertise in communication, conflict resolution, market research, quality assessment, group facilitation, business strategy, and physician relations. Understanding of both the inpatient and outpatient business of women's health is also needed. In essence, the business aspects of the service line should be directed by this role.

Some organizations insist that service line directors have clinical expertise or that a physician or nurse fill the role. Although clinical strength is essential at the point of service and in the direction of operations, integration and business skills are more likely needed for this role rather than clinical expertise. Some health care systems have combined the role of medical director for women's health services with that of the service line director; others designate two directors with overlapping roles. The service line director should emphasize strategic planning, program development, market research and assessment, program coordination and integration, physician relations, business development, and financial accountability for the service line. The medical director for women's health services should be knowledgeable about comprehensive women's health and should possess interpersonal and professional skills similar to that of the service line director. The medical director is responsible for ensuring that quality medical care is available to women through the development of various programs and services throughout the system. Often the role includes strategic planning, policy development, continuing medical education, research and quality improvement, capital equipment planning, and conflict resolution.

Once the organizational structure is defined and positions are delineated, the next step is determining which programs and services should be integrated and which should remain with an entity focus. The next section discusses how these decisions are made and recommends specific programs for women's health that should be considered for integration.

PROGRAM INTEGRATION

Determining which programs and services can be integrated is not easy. As previously mentioned, some positions are aligned to specific programs, and any efforts to consolidate or integrate a program may result in a loss of jobs. To initiate the identification of programs that are candidates for integration, begin with those that will obviously benefit from it.

In one newly formed system, a decision was made to review the breast-feeding education and support services for each hospital and outpatient clinic within the system. Upon completion of the review, it was determined that common elements existed in all of the programs that could easily be integrated, including the orientation and education of new nursing personnel; educational materials provided to new mothers; and consultation referral protocol for patients experiencing difficulties in breast-feeding. A committee of representatives was formed across the system. It developed a mission statement pertaining to the advancement of successful breast-feeding in new mothers. This mission bonded the committee together with a common goal. The next step was to define the elements of a systemwide program for lactation support, education, and consultation. A "system" way of doing things was developed, and every new nurse entering orientation for mother-baby care anywhere in the system was taught the basics of lactation education and support using the same educational materials, policies, and protocol. All education materials developed for patients were standardized. The decision matrix for referral for additional consultation was also developed and implemented in the same manner across the system. Nurses with certification in lactation education or lactation consultation were identified, and the process for referral, documenting the consultation, and providing feedback to the patient's physician was developed.

A billing mechanism for nurse consultation for inpatients and outpatients was also developed and implemented systemwide. The next step was the identification of a physician with the interest, knowledge, and skill to be the system's medical director of lactation services and the final step of referral for the most difficult cases for lactation support.

The development of this systemwide program took approximately eight months from the initial meeting where each entity's program was shared as a "point of information" to the completion of one integrated program for the entire system. The final step was the development of outcome indicators to measure the success of the program, to allow for intersystem comparison, and external benchmarking.

This example demonstrates the synergistic outcomes of integration that results from pooling resources and sharing expertise to accomplish a commonly defined and accepted vision.

Other clinical programs that lend well to integration across the system are those that can share expensive resources such as equipment, professional expertise, promotional materials and advertisement, or educational materials. Examples may include a menopausal education and support programs; osteoporosis education and screening; breast health programs; childbirth preparation and parenting education; infertility programs; perinatology for the management of high-risk pregnancy; and neonatal intensive care.

Clinical programs such as gyn-oncology, urogynecology, infertility, perinatology, and neonatology can be developed in a model similar to regionalized care. In a regional model, one or more hospitals function as the tertiary hospital for the system, and other hospitals provide secondary or Level II care. Patients needing tertiary care are transferred to the tertiary center, or the specialist can rotate through the secondary-system hospitals for consultations and specialized interventions and patient care. This model works particularly well in health care systems where all the hospitals are located within a fairly confined geographical area. The sharing of expensive resources maximizes operational efficiency and enhances the marketability of the systemwide women's health program. Often smaller system hospitals would be unable to afford the specialty services if they were not shared among all system players. The population needed to support the "superspecialties" such as gyn-oncology, urogynecology, and infertility likely could not be achieved in smaller community hospitals unless the needs of the entire system were considered.

In some systems, tertiary hospitals act as hubs for regionalization and should be responsible for providing continuing medical and nursing education and leadership in quality and research initiatives for the entire system. Large systems that are not geographically proximal may also adopt the regional approach to care, but there may be more resistance from physicians and patients to transfer care to a facility some distance from their community. In these cases, the medical specialists may need to establish visiting rotations to the outlying hospitals for specialty consultations.

ORGANIZING A SYSTEMWIDE COUNCIL STRUCTURE

Organizations that foster participative planning and physician partnership need to develop interdisciplinary councils for planning, coordination of programs and services, and integration efforts. One of the first councils needed for the women's service line is the strategic steering council. This committee should include physicians, nurses, and other professionals who represent women's health specialties. Many health care systems develop such a committee but, unfortunately, the membership is largely obstetricians and OB/GYNs, neonatologists or pediatricians, and nurses from the maternal-newborn clinical areas. Although these professionals have knowledge of women's health, it is often from the childbirth or reproductive prospective. For the development of a truly comprehensive women's health service line, the steering committee must be interdisciplinary and multispecialty. Representatives might include physicians and nurses from OB/GYN, family practice with specific interest in women's health, reproductive endocrinology, a fertility specialist, clinical psychology or social services, radiology, and surgeons with specific interest in breast health, community health, and preventive medicine. Another addition might be a specialist (physician, nurse, or other professional) in integrative or complementary therapies. Other specialists can be added when the agenda includes such topics as the development of a systemwide program for gyn-oncology or urogynecology.

The purpose of the steering council is to provide direction to the women's health service line for the development of strategic initiatives; to ensure that quality indicators are developed and expected outcomes are achieved; and to identify programs and services that may need to be added, eliminated, or integrated across the system. In some organizations, all other system committees report at defined times during the year to the steering council, giving an additional oversight responsibility to the council.

Other committees should be developed around integrative needs and initiatives. As an example, if there is a desire to integrate some of the operational aspects of women's services across the system, a systemwide operational council could be developed. This council would be responsible for reviewing operational indicators to ensure financial integrity, patient care quality and satisfaction, staffing efficiency, and professional competence. The operational council might also review capital equipment needs or human resource needs, looking for ways to share expensive resources. In some organizations, this council has also developed consistency across the system in patient documentation systems, nursing orientation and performance standards, patient care policies and procedures, and quality indicators.

Another important council to consider is a research and quality council that could be responsible for identifying the research and quality agenda for the health care system based on quality outcomes, clinical needs, or other research priorities. This council should also be interdisciplinary to ensure consistency among disciplines in research and quality efforts.

A professional development committee is a natural subcommittee for the research and quality council. It would be responsible for ensuring professional competence by standardizing methods to measure professional skills in specific areas, such as fetal and physiological monitoring interpretation or neonatal resuscitation. A continuing education agenda can be developed by this committee annually for both nursing and medicine to expand the knowledge of women's health topics and clinical issues or in response to specific quality concerns.

Many health care systems include a systemwide committee for marketing and business development. Members include system representatives from each entity and the department for corporate planning and marketing. The purpose of this committee is to review current market research data and develop initiatives in program planning, marketing, and promotions, and contracting to build market share in specific programs at each hospital or for the system as a whole.

Other system committees may be program specific and are often developed to coordinate or integrate specific aspects of care. Examples include lactation support, diabetes and pregnancy, preterm birth prevention, and midlife women's health. These committees are often interdisciplinary and chaired by various administrative staff or clinical staff members. Figure 8.6 illustrates one health care system's committee structure to ensure integration of operations, marketing, quality initiatives, and specific program functions.

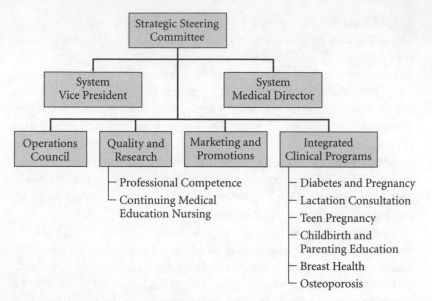

Figure 8.6.   System Committee Structure.

PLANNING FROM A SYSTEM PERSPECTIVE

Strategic planning and program development must occur from the system perspective and must consider the unique needs of each entity within the system. Because each entity must respond to the population needs in the community it serves, the programs and services may differ among entities. The differences are identified and included in the business plan for the service line. Each service and program should be supported with market research data.

One health care system in the Southwest consisted of a tertiary hospital in the central city area and three other hospitals located in suburban areas ten miles apart. Whereas the female population in the center city area was predominantly of childbearing age (eighteen to forty-four years old) and primarily indigent, the suburban hospitals had dramatically different markets. One was located in a community with changing market demographics and with the majority population of women moving into midlife (forty-five to fifty-nine years old). A bimodal population of women of childbearing age and senior women (sixty years and older) surrounded the other two hospitals.

The strategic initiatives for the system would need to include the specific concerns of each of these entities while assessing the impact on the service line as a whole. If the mission were to enhance the market share in women's health services at each of the entities, then population-based planning would indicate the need for different programs and services in each area, and, likely, different marketing and promotional strategies. If the mission were to build volume in deliveries at the tertiary hospital, then a different strategy would be employed for the community hospitals, causing deliveries to be referred to the tertiary hospital for delivery. Apparent in this example is the need to develop clarity and consensus around the strategic mission for the service line so all initiatives can support that outcome.

MARKETING AND PROMOTIONS FROM A SYSTEM PERSPECTIVE

There are many benefits to developing a systemwide approach to marketing and promotions. Advertising dollars can be shared, with system ads promoting the women's health service line rather than any specific hospital or outpatient setting. Collateral materials can be developed promoting the entire system of care for women and eliminating entity-specific collateral material. The entire concept of branding supports the notion that the same level of care in women's services can be received anywhere within the system, and that there is a certain style or philosophy of care that the customer can expect anywhere in it. Many organizations have taken the systemwide approach to marketing and promotions and have achieved savings from it.

Unfortunately, although there are many benefits to the systemwide approach, there are disadvantages as well. If the specific needs of each entity are not considered, target markets may not be reached appropriately. Community-based hospitals may have marketing needs to appropriately package and sell their programs and services to women in defined market sectors, and the collateral and promotional materials may need to be age and market specific to appeal to the targeted audience. Some targeted audiences may not respond to the more generic, corporate advertisement or promotion, but they might be responsive to an entity-based marketing campaign. What is important is that these marketing decisions be made from the system perspective with sensitivity demonstrated at the system level for entity-specific needs.

OUTPATIENT WOMEN'S HEALTH

Most health care systems develop elaborate structures to support specific service line initiatives and inpatient services. The women's health service is somewhat different in that its clinical work is generally performed in a distinct and segregated area of the inpatient setting, but the majority of women's health services are actually provided in an outpatient setting. The service line director must be responsible for integrating outpatient women's services as well. Women's health services can be provided in private physician offices, group practices, clinic settings, women's health centers, freestanding birthing centers, family planning centers, breast centers, employer work sites, chiropractic offices, pharmacies, and other places too numerous to name. All of the outpatient sites sponsored or owned by the health care system should be identified and assessed for quality against a predetermined set of quality standards. More women will be affected by interactions in the outpatient setting than by inpatient encounters.

The health care system's mission for women's health must reach to outpatient settings. It is ideal for the actual mission statement to be posted in outpatient settings specifically for women and should appear in all collateral, promotional, and educational materials used there. A patient satisfaction survey should also be developed to measure women's perceptions of care and satisfaction with the outpatient encounter.

Developing programs and services that will support physicians and other providers in their outpatient women's health practice rather than competing with them is one approach that can be taken by a health care system to advance women's health care in the outpatient setting. As an example, the system might develop menopause or midlife support groups, lactation services, or women's health education at clinic sites or in physician group offices. If the community is devoid of specific screening or diagnostic capabilities such as osteoporosis screening, mammography, lifestyle and fitness appraisal, nutritional assessment and counseling, patient education, or social and behavioral services, these programs should be developed for women at sites that are easily assessable and supportive for the physician's practices.

A health risk appraisal center within a women's health center can be developed and staffed by a nurse practitioner who conducts a health risk appraisal for women on a walk-in basis using a standardized and validated form. Once an issue is identified, the woman who does not have a primary provider can be referred to one covered by her insurance and included on the system's panel. Such a program provides a needed service for women and ensures referrals to the system's providers.

Outpatient care for women should be developed and coordinated from a system perspective as well. An express purpose should be the empowerment of women to become involved in decisions pertaining to their own health and care and to the health of others for whom they are responsible. Clearly, this mission and purpose indicates the necessity for the system to develop support programs to inform, educate, and prepare women for health care decision making, self-care, and care taking. Programs and services in the outpatient setting must include those that promote health and prevent illness through healthy lifestyle maintenance and the early detection of disease through screening and diagnosis. Health care systems that are highly managed and exist in a capitated reimbursement model should be especially interested in the outpatient care and empowerment of women. Because women are the largest consumers of health care in America, keeping them informed, educated, and healthy will reduce expenditures in a prospectively reimbursed system. Other health care systems in a less mature managed care market should realize the benefits of providing excellent outpatient services to women because of the impact on the health and well-being of the total community. As caretakers of the entire family unit, women who are better informed about and prepared for their responsibilities will likely make better decisions to protect their own health and the health of their families.

SUMMARY

The women's health service line plays an important role in newly formed health care systems. The service line provides gender-specific services, but there is considerable overlap with other services, indicating a needed for collaborative strategic planning and program development for women's health services with other lines such as cardiac services, cancer services, behavioral health, and senior health.

With the merging of several hospitals and outpatient settings to form a new organizational unit, a system of care is developed for patients. Many programs and services offered in the women's health service line can be integrated to share expensive resources, reduce duplication of efforts, and expand services in areas void of resources. An organizational structure needs to be developed that will support integration efforts and provide synergistic outcomes that could not be achieved by each entity in the system working independently of one another. By developing integrated systems of care for women, the health care status of women can be greatly improved.

Notes

1. Healy, B. *A New Prescription for Women's Health.* New York: Viking, 1995.
2. American Heart Association. *Your Heart: An Owner's Manual.* Upper Saddle River, N.J.: Prentice Hall, 1995.

CHAPTER NINE

The Social Reconnaissance Approach for Understanding Women's Health

Michael R. J. Felix
James N. Burdine

Michael R. J. Felix is the cofounder of Felix, Burdine & Associates, Inc., an Allentown, Pennsylvania, firm that specializes in improving population and community health status. He has also served as project officer for the Henry J. Kaiser Family Foundation's Health Promotion Initiative.

James N. Burdine, Ph.D., is the cofounder of Felix, Burdine & Associates, Inc. He previously held posts with the American Lung Association and the Research Triangle Institute.

Social Reconnaissance is a process used to assess population health by using multiple data collection methods (such as community discussion groups, analysis of existing health data, and population surveys), in a manner that simultaneously prepares a community for the application of the results of that assessment for population health improvement. This chapter describes the steps in the Social Reconnaissance approach. It describes the types of data collected and how to analyze and integrate it. The process for collecting the data is interactive at the community or grassroots level, and the methodology allows for identification of key issues as well as strategies for their resolution; examples of strategies that have resulted from the Social Reconnaissance are also provided. Examples draw on discussions with more than ten thousand community members across the United States over five years, and a population health survey database consisting of more than twenty thousand individuals who have responded to population health surveys conducted in twenty communities.

THE SOCIAL RECONNAISSANCE APPROACH IN ACTION

An important feature of the approach is the involvement of resource holders in the process of data collection and analysis. A resource holder may be an individual, an organization, or a system (such as a health system) from either the public, private, or philanthropic sectors. They may be internal or external to the community or environment. Resource holders may represent a neighborhood, city, county, region, state or national level; they have time, expertise, energy, money, meeting space, materials, or personnel that can be used to develop or implement health improvement strategies. If resource holders are involved in the data collection process and are established as collaborators with grassroots community representatives who are bound to do something with the information gathered (meaning they are willing to exchange their resources for health improvement), experience suggests that strategies for addressing issues develop simultaneously with data collection.

How does the Social Reconnaissance approach contribute to an understanding of women's health? As demonstrated in previous chapters, women are advocates and decision makers for health care and social services for themselves and their families. Thus, asking them what they need and want is key. Social Reconnaissance (SR) is one way to do that.

An SR session held in November 1998 in Jackson County, Missouri, in the community room of a housing development was attended by about thirty women, most of them single. Many had children, who were passed comfortably from lap to lap. The community meeting had been organized by the Local Investment Commission (LINC), so that a team of representatives from the Health Resources and Services

Administration within the federal Department of Health and Human Services could listen about their health concerns.

The participants were asked to describe their community, the challenges and issues they have in gaining access to health care, the resources available to assist them, and what improvements they would like to see. The only rules governing the discussion were that "all answers are correct" and that everyone should respect each other by listening to what each person had to say. The discussion lasted for ninety minutes.

Themes emerged. The first was how similar the challenges are that these women and their families face in trying to get health care. They described a lack of provider sensitivity to the special needs of single-parent families: "Don't they understand what it took for me to get here in the first place?" "I can't go to a second appointment or pick up a prescription right away." The reasons included a lack of transportation, lack of child care, offices that were open only until 5:00 P.M., and a lack of money or time off from work to do more than make one appointment.

The second theme was that these are challenges for women regardless of their insurance coverage, or lack of it. Several women had income above what is required to qualify for public insurance, yet the jobs they hold offer no health coverage. Some suggested it might be better for their families to be on Medicaid. Others described the sheer frustration, and ultimately fear, of not being able to obtain insurance because of health conditions that made them a risk.

All of these women expressed a desire to lead lives of dignity and respect. They worried out loud for their children and their health. They described their role as the caretaker of the family and themselves, as the person responsible for arranging for health care. They explained how, in their own way, they take the time, energy, and effort to gain knowledge about how to pay for the health care their families need, how to get to the right place at the right time, what they can do in between doctor's visits to keep their family healthy, and how they do all this in the face of a growing sense of being blamed for their situation instead of helped. It is an exhausting job for some.

This is a tremendous opportunity for health care providers (individual practitioners, hospitals, community health centers, health plans, or health systems) to improve both market share and the health status of the population they serve by placing attention on the role of women as advocates and family care managers, and implementing strategies that acknowledge and bolster this role. One way to accomplish this is through community-level strategies that increase access to primary and preventive health services for women, in a way that accounts for the challenges they face and the needs they have (such as child care and transportation) to participate in care. Experience indicates that heightened awareness about services available, improved access to primary and preventive services, and, ultimately, improved health outcomes for the entire population can be achieved by focusing on the role of women as the family health advocate. The SR strategy can provide the information base on which to build approaches for health improvement for women and the entire population, and the process through which strategies surface and are planned and implemented.

UNDERPINNINGS OF THE SOCIAL RECONNAISSANCE

SR is a synthesis of elements from the practice of community organizing, particularly community development. It has evolved from a process that was initially used to determine if communities had desired characteristics for participation in social science research. The community was studied using a set list of health indicators and interviews with key leaders to provide insight and guidance.[1] Among other applications, the Social Reconnaissance has been subsequently used to mobilize a community for health improvement[2] and to determine the best approaches for the funding of community health ideas.[3]

SR places attention first on informing and engaging resource holders in the approach, and then the data collection methods facilitate their interaction with the community. The process also works with local change agents, mobilizes existing resources, and attempts to involve the entire community.

In essence, the approach begins at the top or resource level of an environment and uses population-based qualitative and quantitative data collection tools and organizing strategies to bring resource holders and other community members together to implement health improvement strategies. It is this strategic mix of working with both resource holders as well as grassroots community members and representatives that is a hallmark of the Social Reconnaissance. In addition to involving and engaging resource holders in a population-based approach, maintaining a broader determinant of health vision, leadership, and the enlightened-self interest of resource holders involved in the process also require attention in the Social Reconnaissance.

A broader determinant of health vision is one that recognizes, at the population level, that health is determined largely by income, housing, education, and the environment in which people live and the habits and lifestyle choices they make, but very little by the medical care is available to them.[4] A broader determinant of health vision serves as a license for engaging all sectors of a community in the health improvement process—in the broad view, all have an investment and a contribution to health at the population level. By our definition, community sectors include not for profit agencies and organizations, government, the private sector (business and industry), civic organizations, education, media, the faith community, and philanthropy (as distinct from not-for-profits).

Despite the comparatively small role that medical care may play in the status of a population's health from a broader determinant perspective, health providers (individuals, hospitals, community health centers, health systems, or health plans) or local public health agencies must provide the leadership and energy, and a portion of the resources, for the sustained effort required to improve population health. Some providers complain about being perceived as the "deep pockets" of a community, or as the organization with all the solutions if a leadership position is assumed. However, it is within the mission, and often within the community benefit requirement, for health care providers to fill this role. It is also in their self-interest. As one example of leadership, many providers sponsor a Social Reconnaissance or conduct the process with their own staff.

The tie that binds competing interests in a community together is the concept of enlightened self-interest: achieving individual, organizational, and sectorial interests in the context of a process that is simultaneously working for the greater good of population or community health improvement. Tools like memos of agreement and collaboration contracts can be used to track, monitor, and achieve a match between competing interests.

Consider Lehigh Valley in Pennsylvania. Six competing hospitals used SR to plan, develop, and implement a collaborative local Medicaid health plan. This approach ensured that revenues paid by the state to hospitals and local doctors for care of these patients remained in the Lehigh Valley, instead of funding the administration of a plan outside the community. The benefits to the provider of a local plan are economy of scale for administration, reimbursement, and service delivery, and management of the costs of care for the medically indigent. The benefits to the community include an assurance from providers participating in the plan that excess revenues would be used to fund uninsured children so that they might participate in the plan. In conducting the Social Reconnaissance, then, interests may have to be factored in to implement the data collection methodologies, as well as the strategy that emerges from the process.

THE HOW-TO OF THE SOCIAL RECONNAISSANCE

The steps of SR include defining the purpose; gathering population health information; preparing the briefing packet, organizing, conducting, and processing discussion groups; conducting a population health status survey; analyzing the information gathered in the process; and framing information into reports and follow-ups that lay the groundwork for action. These steps are discussed next in order as they usually occur in real life; however, there are variations and accommodations in this process for local circumstances and constraints. Strategies implemented in follow-up to data gathering and group processing steps are described in this section as the last step of the Social Reconnaissance.

Step 1: Define the Purpose

The purpose will drive the roles, expectations, tasks, time lines, and resources required to implement the remaining steps. Purposes for a Social Reconnaissance have included, among others: to develop partnerships and strategies that can address the needs of uninsured persons; to determine how existing resources can be used to expand access to primary care services for minority or non-English-speaking populations; or to build relationships with state or federal resource holders who have mandates to address health service needs in vulnerable populations, such as migrant farm workers or those infected or affected by HIV/AIDS.

Step 2: Gather Existing Data

The second step is to gather existing population health data for a specified geographic area or population. Operating from a broader determinants' perspective requires the collection of data and information on, for example, demographics, the economy and local income distribution, the education system, state and local policies that influence access to resources, and many other variables.

Much if not all of this data already exists in some form in many communities (and at the state level). Local organizations, such as hospitals or nonprofits that have conducted previous assessments, may also have this information gathered through interviews of key leadership and staff at organizations such as hospitals, health plans, the United Way, or other community organizations.

Organizing these data often involves requesting information from community members, state representatives, or other resource holders. The request-and-exchange process begins to build relationships that will have benefits immediately in the SR process and in the future.

Step 3: Prepare a Briefing Packet

The third step is framing the population health information that has been collected into a document that summarizes and communicates key issues, again from the perspective of the broader determinants. Briefing packets used in a Social Reconnaissance typically include maps highlighting the geographic area of interest, data on key health indicators organized in tables, and text describing demographic, economic, political, social, and cultural information for the area of interest. Particular attention is paid to key trends or themes—for instance, industry and employment trends, population changes, and persistent challenges in accessing services—that might and usually do emerge from the information. The purpose of the briefing packet is to communicate to resource holders some of the challenges and issues a community or state may be facing—in advance of the community discussion process. The document serves as a teaching tool as well: using the briefing packet, resource holders can ask questions during the discussion groups. The briefing packet also helps to initiate discussion among resource holders about roles they might play in strategies that address some of the key issues and trends that emerge from this information.

Step 4: Organize a Series of Discussion Groups

This step describes the setup process for the discussion groups—the most interactive, dynamic, reality-check aspect of the Social Reconnaissance. Community-based intermediaries (defined as organizations or persons who have relationships with, and therefore access to, groups of interest in the assessment process) are involved at this point to organize and manage community discussion groups. In the Jackson County, Missouri, case, LINC used its contacts and networks in public housing, churches, school districts, hospitals, the United Way, local government, and community health centers throughout the region to set up (find a location and provide amenities) and invite (via letter, phone, or personal contact) community members to participate in discussions. Using this approach, over 150 individuals were organized for a series of discussions over two days. In any SR approach, the number and composition of the discussion groups varies based on the purpose of the process, the population of interest, the geographic area to be covered, and the amount of time available to devote to this step. In most cases, a series of ten to twelve meetings over a course of two full days for a county, city, or region under three hundred thousand people is sufficient.

Step 5: Conduct Community Discussion Groups

In this step, community discussion groups are held with a team of resource holders and a facilitator. Resource holders attend community discussion groups that are organized by the community intermediaries into types of meetings: meetings with community leaders, meetings with providers of health and human services, and meetings with citizens. The agenda typically calls for participants to define their community, the challenges they face individually or as a community, the current resources available, advice for addressing issues and challenges, and successful collaborative efforts to address community issues. Questions from resource holders involved in the discussions are also incorporated. The agenda and all the information from the discussion is captured on a flip chart, as well as on a laptop computer if available. This step promotes the ideas and concepts of health by its very public nature.

As a process note, discussion participants usually fill out a sign-in sheet; a final report is made, and possibly a follow-up meeting will be convened by the resource holders to report back the information that has been gathered in the discussion groups. A subtle but important aspect of this step is listening—truly listening—to the participants' health needs, interests, and advice. Listening will facilitate Step 8, which is comparing what was heard with the picture created by the data collected prior to the discussions.

Step 6: Process the Experience

The discussion group experience is processed with resource holders during formal briefing sessions held at the conclusion of the discussion group process. During facilitated briefing sessions conducted after the discussion groups, resource holders participating in the strategy offer what they observe to be key themes, health issues, and trends that have emerged from the data collected. Preliminary ideas, opportunities, recommendations, and next steps to address these issues are discussed. This step helps to decipher roles and opportunities that all members of a community or system—including resource holders—can play in the health improvement process. Although the concept of enlightened self-interest is at play throughout the Social Reconnaissance, the briefing sessions serve as the place where interest becomes positioned and used as the rationale for why resource holders from various sectors have a role in follow-up strategies.

Step 7: Conduct a Population Health Status Survey

The population health status survey is implemented after the community discussion groups. During that step, for example, you often learn about language translations that need to be made available, and who in the community can do an appropriate translation of the English-version survey. You also learn about particular issues that might require new questions to be developed and incorporated into the survey document. Use an instrument that has been tested and validated and a methodology that has yielded high response rates across many different types of communities.[5]

The survey data complement the data that already exist in the community, but the survey may also provide new data, such as on functional health status measures or community satisfaction with health and human services that have not been available previously.

Step 8: Analyze and Report the Data

In this step, analyze and report the data collected from the discussion groups and the survey. Prior to writing the discussion group report, the verbatim comments collected during the meetings are analyzed for themes and trends, and the information is then summarized in the order of the discussion group agenda: issues, challenges, resources, existing collaborative efforts, and advice from the participants. To complement these summary points, detailed findings from each discussion group are part of the report. Special attention is paid to presenting the purpose for the discussion groups, and acknowledging the community intermediaries in the process.

The report is the first step in follow-up to the SR: it offers feedback to the community about what was learned and ideas that emerged and suggests roles, opportunities, and next steps that can be played by the resource holders in collaboration with the community. Often, meetings are convened to distribute the report, and press conferences or kick-off meetings to address issues are held in conjunction with such an event.

Data from the general population survey is also reported at this point in the process separately or in a document that presents the findings from all data collection methods conducted in the Social Reconnaissance. Because the data collection process for the survey is lengthier than the community discussion group process, there may be a few weeks or months between Steps 7 and 8.

Step 9: Follow Up

Advice solicited from discussion group participants serves as the basis for follow-up from the initial information-gathering efforts. The strategies and roles for the various resource holders discussed during the briefing sessions can often be paired with this advice to create a powerful recommended course of action. Advice from the discussion groups has included guidance for specific organizations or entities: for example, "The state could provide us with summary information on select health status indicators." State representatives may be part of the team and realize that they have data that would be useful for the community.

All of these steps work together to bring resource holders and the community to a place where strategies that can improve population health are implemented.

CONDUCTING A SOCIAL RECONNAISSANCE

Who can conduct a Social Reconnaissance? When should it be done in a community, state, or region? To the first question, keep in mind that the steps in the Social Reconnaissance are described here from an outsider's point of view: that is, from the viewpoint of those who play a coordination, facilitation, or data collection role in the process. Any institution, organization, or person can play such a role. What changes is the perspective of who is an external rather than an internal resource holder. For example, if a community health center is sponsoring a Social Reconnaissance, external resource holders might include foundations or state associations. If a state is conducting a Social Reconnaissance, outside resource holders might include foundations, as well as federal representatives.

When should a Social Reconnaissance be conducted? SR can be conducted at any stage of a population health improvement process. The approach can be used to gather ideas that a new community health partnership can tackle, or discover and organize commitments from existing resources prior to the implementation of a program that is designed to address an already identified community issue. It can be used, with its combination of qualitative or quantitative approaches, to evaluate strategies that have already been implemented. In this sense, it is a flexible approach, and ultimately tailored to each purpose within the framework described here.

DATA AND THE SOCIAL RECONNAISSANCE

The Social Reconnaissance seeks to frame an understanding of the health of a population within broader determinants of health vision.[6] This understanding requires that issues like income, education, and housing become major considerations in understanding the health process. Ignoring the role income plays for many in our country, especially for women, leaves out valuable information that can help us better design local approaches. For example, many low-income women cannot afford to purchase health insurance or to pay the coinsurance or deductibles for health services that are not covered. Many elect to remain uninsured because it means a higher paycheck. Poverty often prevents women from seeking and receiving the health care they and their families need.

Attention must be directed to the psychological, political, social, and cultural considerations in a population. From a psychological perspective, the pressures faced by single female parents—providing food, shelter, clothing, and arranging for child care and transportation while often lacking emotional support—are important factors that must both be understood and incorporated in health improvement strategies.[7]

This perspective drives the types of data required for the Social Reconnaissance, the places and sources that data are gathered from, as well as the data analysis approach. The importance of both of these aspects warrants further description.

Data Sources

Briefly, sources include secondary and existing data, population health status surveys, and community discussion group data.

Secondary and existing data. An important dimension of collecting data that already exist on the health of a geographic area or population of interest is the use of local contact people and organizations to help assemble the data. For example, a local hospital may have recently completed an assessment that has information on the prevalence of disease in the community, and particular insight about how and where to collect utilization statistics for use of health services. The Chamber of Commerce most likely has a list of the top ten employers by industry. To make the process manageable, a list of sources available and a strategy for their assembly is organized in the second step of the Social Reconnaissance.

Requesting data and information from organizations or individuals requires explaining the purpose for your request and what will be done with it. This request-exchange process builds relationships that allow other partners into the SR process.

Nonlocal sources for information might include the U.S. Census Bureau, Centers for Disease Control (CDC) Wonder database, national and state Behavioral Risk Factor Survey data, and other data obtainable from state Web sites (including from state departments of health). Web-based federal sources of data can be accessed as well.

Population health status surveys. The population health survey utilized in SR gathers data on access to health and human services (including barriers to access), consumer satisfaction with primary care services, functional health status, diseases and disabilities, behavioral risk factors, insurance coverage, and basic demographics.

Questions in the current Felix, Burdine and Associates' survey instrument have their origins in the Medical Outcomes Study, the Centers for Disease Control and Prevention Behavioral Risk Factor Surveillance Survey (CDC-BRFSS), the Primary Care Assessment Survey,[8] and the original Group Health Association of America Consumer Satisfaction Survey. The SF-12 functional health status instrument is a component of each of the community surveys, and has been incorporated for its promise in measuring health status improvement at the individual and population level.[9] All other elements were developed by the firm in conjunction with the communities that have participated in population health status surveys since 1992.

Population health surveys have many benefits beyond gathering timely, firsthand data, which is specific for the population of interest. We have found opportunity for health providers and facilities to more adequately address accreditation, community benefit, or evaluation needs by conducting population health surveys. For example, in Fort Collins, Colorado, the Poudre Health Services District (PHSD) conducted a population-based health assessment using a survey and discussion groups in 1995. Based on that data, services were developed by PHSD and implemented in the community. In 1998, the district conducted a second survey, using a similar instrument (and a discussion group process) to measure overall changes in health status and to evaluate the impact of programs that were developed to address issues identified in the first survey, such as the need for prescription assistance.

The Social Reconnaissance as an entire strategy, particularly the population health status assessment component, has been used by health care providers to demonstrate how they are assessing community needs; this demonstration contributes to meeting both JCAHO requirements for community needs assessment as well as community benefit standards that must be met according to state or local regulations. SR has also been used to understand the entire health care marketplace in a region, with the data subsequently applied for strategic planning of health services.

There are additional key elements that have an impact on population health status—such as the trust among people, social supports available in an environment or to an individual, level of involvement in a community—that are now capable of being measured for their relationship to the health of a population. Researchers around the country are developing measures and measurement techniques to capture the concept of "social capital,"[10] and these can be incorporated into population surveys as well as the community discussion group and observation process. This area of study holds great promise for generating a range of nontraditional strategies that might be recommended for improving population health. Programs and activities that increase the trust and involvement of community members are now legitimately in the realm of health improvement.

Community discussion group data. Information gathered from community discussions is qualitative and consists of perceptions of critical issues and challenges. Referring back to the agenda typically used for a community discussion, the discussion group findings also yield a database of community resources, community contacts and key individuals, and a list of collaborative efforts that can be built on when future health improvement strategies are implemented.

Analysis Approach

One approach to the analysis and application of the data resulting from a Social Reconnaissance is to develop profiles of the population based on factors such as demographics, utilization patterns, insurance status, and functional health status. Local interest helps drive what profiles are developed; for example, the Medicaid or Medicare insured population is often of interest, as are racial, ethnic, and cultural groups.

When developing profiles, try to draw information from all data sources. With an integrated data set, you can compare qualitative and quantitative measures of the same idea or health indicator. For example, you can compare trends in infant mortality with the perception of community members on the seriousness or prominence of infant deaths in the community. You can also compare state estimates of the proportion of adults who are Medicaid enrolled, similar estimates by health providers in the community, and the proportion of persons who are Medicaid insured according to a general population survey. You can compare state or county estimates of the proportion of non-English-speaking children in elementary schools with the proportion cited by school principals for current enrollment, and estimate the proportion of cultural or ethnic groups in a population based on survey responses.

It is often possible to compare issues across the community using qualitative data. For example, access to care may be perceived as a challenge by health and human service providers as well as consumers. Comparing data at different levels of specificity can also provide important insights. For example, county-level data are often available for population estimates by income, race, or ethnicity. Looking within a county, at a municipality, or in the service area of a provider that crosses municipalities usually demonstrates that county values mask dramatically different rates and experiences for pockets or groups (like a municipality) within the population. The profiling approach recognizes that there may be significant variations for particular groups, and attempts to capture these differences.

As an additional resource to conduct comparative analyses, the survey components from over a dozen Social Reconnaissance projects have been assembled into the Community Health Studies Database. This database can be used to compare survey data collected in any community with others that are similar in size or rural, urban, or suburban nature; a national sample; or with estimates from the entire database. The communities represented range from a single city to a multicounty area, and they are a mix of rural, suburban, and urban areas. Each community has contributed approximately fifteen to eighteen hundred respondents to the database, and there are a total number of 21,458 respondents available for analysis.

REACHING WOMEN: ACCESS TO PRIMARY AND PREVENTIVE CARE

Women are the consumer advocates for families. Learning about that role in a population-based process such as the Social Reconnaissance, and building strategies that subsequently reach women across all economic and cultural boundaries, gives access to an entire population and fosters and builds on the momentum being created by consumer choice to increase market share.[11] Improving access to primary medical care and preventive health services is key to reaching this market.

Women's Access

Listen to women in community discussions and you will hear many reasons for lack of access to primary care. These reasons include being uninsured or not having a regular primary care physician. The cost of wellness visits not covered by insurance may be beyond a family's budget. Women who are employed indicate that lack of after-hours care is one reason they do not have access, particularly if jobs do not permit them to take time off during the day or if they commute significant distances from their home community where the family physician is located. Lack of transportation is a universal challenge, and it comes in many forms: not having a reliable car or any car at all, no public transportation or taxis, or costs for public transportation that are outside the economic means of the family. For medical visits when a woman needs to be seen alone, such as for an annual OB/GYN exam, not having child care can be a barrier. For women who are single parents, these challenges are compounded.

The following groups of people indicate that their overall access to primary care is "poor" or "fair:"

- Persons with children from six to seventeen years of age in the home rate their access as poor or fair more frequently than persons who have no children or only children under age six.

- Persons employed full-time and full-time homemakers rate their access as poor or fair more frequently than those who are employed part-time, are unemployed, are retired, or are students.

- Persons aged thirty-five to forty-four and forty-five to fifty-four tend to rate their access as poor or fair more frequently than those aged eighteen to thirty-four, fifty-five to sixty-four, sixty-five to seventy-four, or seventy-five and older.

- Persons with less than a high school diploma rate their access as poor or fair more frequently than those who are high school or college educated.

- Persons with low incomes (between 100 and 200 percent of the poverty level) rated their access as poor or fair more frequently than those with incomes at or below 100 percent of the poverty level or with incomes at or above 200 percent of the poverty level.

- Persons who are uninsured rate their access as poor or fair more frequently than persons with any type of insurance (Medicare, Medicaid, or commercial insurance). In fact, the largest proportion of households with no health insurance is those with a single, female head of household with dependent children.

Gender may not be statistically related to poor access to care; however, these data complement what is often heard in community discussions. Full-time employed women may have a more difficult time arranging for primary care. Women with young children may in fact have poor access because of a lack of child care. Persons with lower incomes, even if insured, may lack the immediate cash resources to pay for services that are not covered by insurance. Employment, family composition and needs, and income must all be factored into strategies that attempt to increase access to services for women.

Preventive screenings are an important aspect of women's health and could be a higher priority for them if it were available at minimal cost (covered by insurance plans, or if preventive services were free or at low cost), or if some preventive care and education was provided when women do interact with the system for other family members: when they have a sick child who needs a check up, or an infant being seen for regular care. Workplace or neighborhood locations for screenings and education have been suggested as ways to address multiple barriers to accessing preventive care.

In the Community Health Studies database, data on preventive health screenings by women, specifically to detect cancers (such as clinical breast exams, Pap smears, and mammograms), can provide insight on the opportunity for outreach to women via preventive health approaches. Using the Community Health Studies database, we have tried to estimate the opportunity for outreach by analyzing the proportion and types of women who have never had recommended preventive screenings. For this analysis, summarized in Table 9.1, community survey respondents are placed in the following categories:

- Four race and ethnicity categories: black, Hispanic/Latino, white, and other

- Three income categories: poverty (income under 100 percent of the federal poverty level), low income (between 101 percent and 200 percent of the poverty level), and above low income (more than 200 percent of the poverty level)

- Six age groups: eighteen to thirty-four, thirty-five to forty-four, forty-five to fifty-four, fifty-five to sixty-four, sixty-five to seventy-four, and seventy-five and older

- Three categories of educational attainment: less than a high school diploma, high school graduate, and some college or vocational education

- Four "household type" groups: males (married or unmarried), married females, single females with no children, and single females with children. These categories were specifically designed to highlight women who serve as the head of a household, as distinct from married women.

A higher proportion of Latino/Hispanic and black women respondents reported never having had a mammogram, a clinical breast exam, or a Pap smear than whites or others. Women with a total household

Never having a screening most frequently reported by:	Race/ Ethnicity	Income	Age Groups	Educational Attainment	Household Type
Never Had a Breast Exam	Latino/ Hispanic	Poverty	18–34, 75+	Less than high school diploma	Single female, single female with child(ren)
Never Had a Pap Smear	Latino/ Hispanic, African-American	Poverty	18–34, 75+	Less than high school diploma	Single female with child(ren)
Never Had a Mammogram	—	Poverty	—	Less than high school diploma	Single female with child(ren)

Table 9.1.   Demographic Groups Reporting Never Having Types of Preventive Health Screenings.

income at or below the federal poverty level and single women (both with and without children) were more likely to report never having preventive screenings than women with incomes above 100 percent of the poverty level or women who are married. Although mammography has age-specific guidelines for screening, both Pap smears and breast exams are part of normal routine care for women age eighteen and over.

Strategies for Improving Access

There are opportunities for resource holders to improve access to primary and preventive services for women, including the following:

1. Implementing and communicating policy statements at the board level of an organization that acknowledge the significant role women play as family health advocates. The first step here is using population-based health information to ensure that board members, administrative personnel, providers, payors, and the community from which any information is collected are aware of what those data mean. The second step is engaging them in determining what should be acted on based on the information gathered. This education process sets the stage for making the necessary adjustments in other aspects of the health system.

2. Lack of culture and language sensitivity is often a barrier to receiving appropriate health care. Planning and implementing visible protocols (such as signs in Spanish indicating how to call for an interpreter) that promote an appreciation and understanding of cultural differences assures consumers of the provider's interest in removing barriers. This sensitivity may require training, education, and tech nical assistance programs for staff that address cultural values and language differences. Literacy and language education programs for women and their families is the companion to this approach: many communities have programs in place where health care providers can participate as partners in literacy programs. Where these programs do not exist, leadership calls for health care providers to help plan, organize, and implement these activities.

3. Instead of traditional 9 to 5 and some evening hours, suggestions from women for ideal hours of operation range from 12 to 9 Monday through Saturday to facilities that are open in shifts. Each community has its own set of conditions that might drive optimal hours. The point is that working women have little opportunity to get care during more traditional hours. Making adjustments could improve the situation easily.

4. Lack of understanding and knowledge about health, or lack of knowledge about the range and type of services available, hampers consumers' ability to make decisions.[12] Providers, too, lack information about the availability of other community resources that may be engaged to support women in the health process. Implementing community approaches to improve women's knowledge of available health services (such as information hotlines and one-stop places for service information) can yield major health improvement opportunities and more appropriate use of services. Community health education strategies that use traditional media such as newspapers, newsletters, television, and radio, as well as the more sophisticated communication strategies that, for example, connect World Wide Web health resources (such as libraries or research articles) to local community library kiosks provide a wide variety of health and service information.

5. Lack of child care and transportation are issues that women face as they attempt to gain access to health and human services in their neighborhoods and cities. Health care providers that begin to factor these considerations into their process for delivering services—such as by providing child care, transportation to and from services, or after-hours care—will make major strides toward engaging women.

SOCIAL RECONNAISSANCE: CASE STUDIES

In Perth Amboy, New Jersey, SR was convened by the Jewish Renaissance Foundation, an organization seeking ways to better serve the low-income and uninsured members of its community. One issue that surfaced during the Social Reconnaissance (which consisted of discussion groups and secondary data gathering) was lack of access to primary medical care, including prenatal care for women, particularly for the Hispanic population. The need for improved communication and increased awareness on the part of both service providers and community members around what services are available in the community was also identified.

Several follow-up strategies are in motion as part of the Social Reconnaissance. The foundation is using the Social Reconnaissance report as a reason to reconvene participants from the community discussion groups, as well as other community resource holders to communicate the results of the information gathering process and to organize task groups that address the need for centralized, coordinated information and the need for primary care services. As one solution, the foundation is marshaling its resources to expand the hours of a local hospital-based clinic to increase access by providing after-hours services and to recruit Spanish-speaking providers that can meet the special needs of the dominant Hispanic population in the city, particularly for Hispanic women.

In Augusta, Georgia, the Social Reconnaissance helped to bring to the community's attention the many challenges that low-income and working poor persons have in accessing primary care. The assessment process isolated a zip code in the city that contained a high proportion of poor residents, a high incidence of violent events and reported emotional problems by community members, limited access to transportation, uses of the emergency room for care, and a high proportion of uninsured persons. The Augusta hospitals and the health department formed a partnership that implemented a primary-care center in a Baptist church. This center was created to specifically serve individuals located within the 30901 zip code of Augusta. Since then, the partnership has expanded this model of primary care delivery to other zip codes, and has brokered additional human services and health promotion programs into these centers for the communities they serve.

SUMMARY

This chapter describes a strategy that is gaining popularity as a means of understanding the health status of individuals and populations and using this knowledge to plan and implement local health improvement strategies.

The Social Reconnaissance methods—population surveys, community discussion groups, and analysis of secondary data—have yielded important consumer suggestions and subsequent strategies for improving health status and increasing market share. These methods have brought to light the needs of entire communities and of special groups within a community. Women have been identified as one of these groups, not only because of their own health needs and issues, but because of the role they play in advocating for the health of themselves and their families.

The challenges for health providers and payers are both the adoption of useful health status information-gathering strategies such as the Social Reconnaissance and the application of the information gathered in ways that recognize the consumer advocacy role women are playing. This may involve retooling local policy, administrative, financing, and service delivery mechanisms to appropriately capitalize on this role. The beauty of this type of approach, focused on women, is that it will cut across lines of race, ethnicity, economics, and geography to reach an entire population of people that includes men and children.

Health providers and systems that collect, analyze, and apply local health status information in strategies such as those suggested in this chapter to specifically meet the needs and interests of women can benefit in several areas:

- Product or provider loyalty or relationships can be established that, over time, can and should have a favorable impact on both the health status of women and families and improve the bottom line and market share. The influence of these loyalties will be more important as consumer preferences begin to drive choice of health care providers and even shape health plan benefits.[13]

- The leadership opportunities for health facilities and providers in the strategies suggested in this chapter are consistent with the community benefit requirements of not-for-profit entities, particularly those in health care. For-profit entities also can improve community relations and enhance marketing opportunities through these approaches—all of which can have an impact on market share.

The most important aspect of the Social Reconnaissance is the opportunity it creates for listening to people. Listening leads to recognition that consumer health advocacy is becoming an important part of the health process. Strategies to reach women, such as those that improve access to primary and preventive services, cut across all boundaries and can lead to health status improvement for the entire population—as well as improved market share for providers. The Social Reconnaissance is an effective tool for helping communities understand these related opportunities.

Notes

1. Sanders, I. T. "The Community Social Profile." *American Sociological Review,* 1975, *25,* 75–77; Sanders, I. T. "The Social Reconnaissance Method of Community Study." In H. K. Schwarzweller (ed.), *Research in Rural Sociology and Development: Focus on Community.* Vol. 2. Greenwich, Conn.: JAI Press, 1985.

2. Stunkard, A. J., Felix, M.R.J., and Cohen, R. Y. "Mobilizing a Community to Promote Health: The Pennsylvania County Health Improvement Program (CHIP)." In J. C. Rosen and L. J. Solomon (eds.), *Prevention in Health Psychology.* Hanover, N.H.: University Press of New England, 1985; Felix, M.R.J. "The Partnership Approach for Sustaining Heart Health." *Canadian Journal of Cardiology,* 1993, *9* (suppl. D), 165D–167D.

3. Tarlov, A., and others. "Foundation Work: The Health Promotion Program of the Henry J. Kaiser Family Foundation." *American Journal of Health Promotion,* 1987, *2,* 74–80;Williams, R. M. "Rx: Social Reconnaissance." *Foundation News,* 1990, *31,* 24–29.

4. World Health Organization. *The Constitution of the World Health Organization.* Geneva, Switzerland: World Health Organization, 1948; Ontario Health Review Panel. *Toward a Shared Direction for Health in Ontario.* Toronto, Canada: Ontario Health Review Panel, 1987.

5. Burdine, J. N., and others. "The SF-12 as a Population Health Measure: Potential for Application." Unpublished manuscript, 1998.

6. World Health Organization, *Constitution;* Ontario Health Review Panel, *Toward a Shared Direction.*

7. Tarlov, A., and Felix, M.R.J. "The Production of Health in America: Mobilizing Communities." Unpublished manuscript, 1993; Tarlov, A. "The Coming Influence of a Social Sciences Perspective on Medical Education." *Academic Medicine,* 1992, *67,* 722–729.

8. Safran, D. G., and others. "The Primary Care Assessment Survey: Tests of Data Quality and Measurement Performance." *Medical Care,* 1998, *36,* 728–739.

9. Burdine and others, "The SF-12"; Ware, J. E., Kosinski, M., and Keller, S. D. *SF-12: How to Score the SF-12 Physical and Mental Health Summary Scales.* Boston: Health Institute, New England Medical Center, 1995.

10. Lomas, J. "Social Capital and Health: Implications for Public Health and Epidemiology." *Social Science and Medicine,* 1998, 9, 1181–1188.

11. KPMG. "The New Challenge for Health Care Leaders: Using Consumer Focus to Improve Revenue Management and Sustain Organizational Growth." Educational Series, 1998.

12. KPMG. "Consumerism in Health Care: New Voices." *Consumerism in Health Care Research Study Findings,* Jan. 1998.

13. Llewellyn, A., Burdine, J. N., and Felix, M.R.J. "Managed Care and Mental Health Services: Implications for the Consumer." *Journal of the California Alliance for the Mentally Ill,* 1996, 7, 19–21.

CHAPTER TEN

The Underserved Woman as a Business Consideration

Genie James
Stacy A. Graham
Laura J. Reed

> *Stacy A. Graham is a marketing and communications consultant in Stayton, Oregon. She is currently advocate for community mobilization, collaboration, and outcomes-based programming for the Oregon Commission on Children and Families and a member of the Coordinating Team of Friends of the Family, a locally based nonprofit organization serving four communities in rural Oregon.*

> *Laura J. Reed is a Nashville-based writer who also serves as a consultant to hospitals and health management and health information companies.*

Executives making financial decisions for today's health care organizations tend to prioritize ideas in terms of revenue streams. Those who do not see underserved populations as a source of revenue may be tempted to dismiss this chapter. But first, they should calculate the financial impact of what happens when these populations are ignored. Developing a pro forma that covers common primary care and preventive services is usually less expensive in the long run than having to pay for the more intensive, invasive, or long-term treatments that become necessary when primary care and prevention are neglected.

A critical strategic issue facing health care leaders today is improving the efficiency with which they address the needs of the uninsured and underserved. Using a Census Bureau database, the Health Insurance Association of America recently found that under current economic conditions more than fifty-three million nonelderly people in the United States, or more than one out of five people, will be uninsured by 2007.[1] The number of uninsured—most of them women—is growing steadily. Previous chapters have made clear why women and their needs deserve your attention. This chapter focuses on the uninsured and underserved woman. A few facts illuminate why this attention is important:

- With managed care, capitation, and decreasing Medicaid and Medicare reimbursements, providers are already asked to do more for less when treating this population subset. This trend is not likely to reverse itself.

- The demand for services among underserved women will only continue to increase. Women of the baby-boom generation, who already represent a majority of both Medicaid and Medicare enrollees, will require the higher levels of health care associated with aging and chronic illness.

- Medicare beneficiaries over age sixty-five with incomes below the federal poverty level but still eligible for Medicaid—most of whom are women—spent 35 percent of their income on health care; those who were not eligible for Medicaid assistance spent half their incomes on health care.[2]

As with any population subset, the basic business principle of supply and demand has an impact on service delivery. When faced with increasing demand and decreasing reimbursement, health care providers must become more efficient and proactive in their services delivery. Primary care, health education, health risk screening, and early detection and treatment never made more sense than with this population. Indeed, a wealth of program case studies document improvements in health status through community-level programs, some of which, despite the complexity of the confounding variables and a lack of funding for studies, have quantified related savings.[3] Evidence of the cost-effectiveness of prevention is available in numerous studies of corporate health promotion programs, which not only reveal that such efforts can yield significant improvements in health status but also positive return-on-investment ratios.[4]

Still, many hospital CEOs dismiss strategies targeting the poor as largely public relations efforts or as admirable but not necessary charitable initiatives aimed at giving back to the community. But when health care for the poor is paid for by the hospitals' most prominent payor, the government, these same executives had better change their mind-set. In developing a business strategy to meet the needs of the underserved, in short, will you pay now or pay later? Doing nothing is not an option. The costs of care can multiply when primary care is delivered in the emergency room. Providing for the needs of the underserved is not only a key mission of most hospitals and health systems, it is also a financially sound endeavor that providers simply cannot afford to neglect.

The problem of developing cost-effective and efficient services for the underserved is vast and complex. Thus health care executives need to take the practical approach. They first must identify key information needed to make informed decisions:

- Who are the underserved in the community?
- What do they want and need?
- How can services be delivered most effectively to them?

These are the questions addressed in this chapter.

UNDERSTANDING YOUR CUSTOMER

To really know the underserved in your community, spend some time in the unemployment office. Sign up as a volunteer through a church or United Way and go where they need you most. Visit local Head Start classrooms and those sections of your city that you don't dare frequent alone or at night. The next sections may help prepare you for what you'll see.

Poverty, Women, and Medicaid

Overall, 13.3 percent of Americans were below the poverty level in 1997. Of those, 23 percent were adult women and 40 percent were children. Some states (Mississippi and New Mexico) and the District of Columbia then had poverty levels exceeding 20 percent; a dozen were in the high teens. These numbers are significant. Table 10.1 shows how the federal government defines poverty.

Providers must take note of these statistics because they tie clients to a major source of managed care revenue and Medicaid reimbursement. Since the mid-sixties, Medicaid has provided health care coverage to the poorest of the poor; in recent years it has expanded to allow states to extend Medicaid coverage to those with incomes well above the federal poverty level.[5]

More recently, the Children's Health Insurance Program (CHIP) has continued this trend. It grew out of the Balanced Budget Act of 1997, when Congress set a goal to reduce the number of uninsured children from ten million to two million by 2002. Though the program is making progress, it is plagued by the inherent problems of adequately reaching those eligible and making them, and providers, aware of the programs.[6] Public-private sector collaborative efforts have helped some states boost enrollment.[7]

The Improved Maternal and Children's Health Coverage Act of 1999, before Congress in the spring of 1999, would expand coverage to additional immigrant children and require states to coordinate enrollment between Medicaid, CHIP, and other programs, as well as to participate in a national toll-free information line.[8] This could have a direct impact on the distribution of funds at the local level.

Size of Family	Weighted Average Threshold
One person	$8,183
Under 65	$8,350
65+	$7,698
Two people	$10,473
Householder Under 65	$10,805
Householder 65+	$9,712
Three people	$12,802
Four people	$16,400
Five people	$19,380
Six people	$21,886
Seven people	$24,802
Eight people	$27,593
Nine people	$32,566

Table 10.1.   Government Poverty Thresholds, 1997.
Source: U.S. Bureau of the Census.

Managed care penetration into Medicaid will undoubtedly have its own effect. Already 15.3 million Medicaid enrollees are in some sort of managed care plan. More time is needed to accurately measure the effect of this change on access, quality, and use of preventive services, but some early studies suggest positive results.[9] Arizona began managing its Medicaid programs early on and has documented savings of 7 to 11 percent annually accompanied by high levels of patient satisfaction.[10] This program has already become a model for other states' efforts.

Medicaid and women's health are intrinsically linked. Fifty-eight percent of Medicaid enrollees are female. In June 1999, nearly 203,000 women were enrolled in Medicaid (see Table 10.2). As a percentage of the U.S. population, 15 percent of U.S. women use Medicaid compared to 10 percent of men. The racial distribution of Medicaid enrollees is not consistent with that of the nation as a whole (see Figure 10.1). The age distribution raises the question of how—or if—the poor in the middle age groups are receiving their health care.

Low-Income Americans and the Uninsured

According to research by Tatiana Masters and Cathy Lindenberg at the University of Washington School of Nursing, a woman is more likely to be poor than a man, and poor women are disproportionately racial or ethnic minorities. The majority of poor adult women are in their childbearing years—between eighteen and forty-four years old.

Even college-educated women earn less than men. And despite the success many women have recently achieved as business executives, women who hold the same positions as men still often earn significantly less.

For many of the working poor, the choice is between health care and food on the table. Nationwide, 14.8 percent of all women and 28.4

Age	Number of Females	Percentage of Females
0–6	38,605	19.03
7–18	42,946	21.17
19–44	70,166	34.59
45–64	27,335	13.48
65+	23,777	11.72
Total	202,826	100.00

Table 10.2.   Distribution of Medicaid Enrollment: Females by Age, 1999.
Source: Medicaid Eligibility Files, June 1999.

percent of poor women had no health insurance in 1997. The highest uninsured rate was among women and men of Hispanic origin (34.2 percent) and people of foreign birth (34.3 percent). Poor immigrants are in the worst position: 51 percent were without coverage. The Department of Commerce reports that in 1997, 43.4 million Americans (16.1 percent) had no health care coverage of any kind for the entire calendar year. Of those, 14.8 percent were women and 28.4 percent were poor women. Among the general population eighteen to sixty-four years old, workers were more likely to be insured than nonworkers, but among the poor the opposite is true.[11]

The Forgotten Women

The numbers don't tell the whole story. Typically forgotten or overlooked in the data are at least three groups: single women, lesbians, and female migrant workers.

In 1999, the National Law Center on Homelessness and Poverty estimated that about two million people are homeless.[12] Single women are about 14 percent of the urban homeless population. Families with children account for 40 percent of the homeless and are among the fastest-growing segments of the homeless population. In its 1998 survey of 30 cities, the U.S. Conference of Mayors found that domestic violence was a primary cause of homelessness, and that the homeless population was 53 percent black, 35 percent white, 12 percent Hispanic, 4 percent Native American and 3 percent Asian. A study in New York City found that homelessness is associated with substantial excess costs per hospital stay.[13]

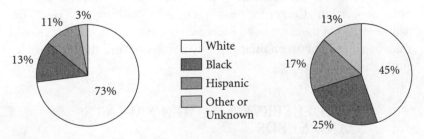

Figure 10.1. Racial and Ethnic Distribution Compared to Medicaid Enrollees, 1996.

Source: U.S. Bureau of the Census.

A group that has gained increasing prominence is migrant workers. Every year in America, between three and five million migrant and seasonal farm workers harvest crops. Typically working as families, 80 percent of them are Latinos and 63 percent are legally authorized to work in the United States. They are in need; their average annual income is less than $7,500; 70 percent live below the poverty level; and on average they have six years of schooling. The special health problems they experience due to their dismal working and housing conditions are many: high rates of accidents, pesticide poisoning, urinary tract and other infections, dehydration, heat stroke, diabetes, hypertension, tuberculosis, psychosocial stress, and depression. In many cases they are eligible for Medicaid and Aid to Families with Dependent Children, but most are unable to register for such services due to their mobile status or are unaware of the programs entirely. Migrant health centers have the capacity to serve fewer than 15 percent of them. But because migrants do not receive sick leave and are afraid of losing wages, they often do not attempt to obtain the services available to them.[14]

Looking Ahead

The problem of the underserved is likely to worsen in the coming years, especially for women. By 2010, one-third of the female population living alone will be between the ages of forty-five and sixty-four, so Medicare will not yet be available to them. Some of these women may have to resort to other programs such as Medicaid, and it will be each state's responsibility to decide how to provide services. "We are doing pretty well around the country with services for reproductive health, breast cancer and cervical cancer," noted Joan Henneberry, program director for Maternal and Child Health at the National Governors Association's Center for Best Practices in Washington, D.C. "The bad news is that there are not a lot of programs or service dollars available for women between their reproductive years and the time of eligibility for Medicare."[15]

UNDERSERVED WOMEN'S WANTS AND NEEDS

A focus group of fifty low-income women of diverse ethnic backgrounds revealed few differences when asked about their expectations from their prenatal care provider. They valued the following:[16]

- The technical competence of the practitioner
- The continuity of care
- The atmosphere and physical environment of the care setting

Another study, conducted among black and Hispanic Medicaid recipients, found similar results: "having the procedure explained by the provider" was the most important determinant of satisfaction for both groups.[17] Not surprisingly, both studies found that low-income women want what we all want: good care, well explained. They also want the health care community to help keep them healthy and well. They want an emphasis on preventive medical services for themselves and their families.

Because underserved women are more likely to be poor, and their access to health care further limited by language and cultural barriers, discussions of their health status are to a large extent discussions of the health status of minority women. The 26 percent (thirty-five million) of Americans who are minority women experience most of the same health problems as others in the nation, but their health outcomes are poorer than those of Caucasian women.[18] For example:

- Black women have higher death rates than white women from two of the leading causes of death, heart disease and stroke. Their mortality rates are higher from most cancers, HIV/AIDS, homicide, alcohol, and drug-induced causes.

- Asian and Pacific Islander women have higher death rates from injuries and suicide than white women.

- American Indian and Alaska native women have higher death rates from diabetes and cirrhosis of the liver than white women.[19]

- 1996 data show that 71.3 percent of black women, 66.7 percent of American Indian and Alaska native women, and 71.9 percent of Hispanic women receive early prenatal care. These figures are better than in the past, but a gap remains. Between 1987 and 1996, the number of women receiving first-trimester prenatal care in America increased from 76 percent to 81.8 percent.

- Breast-feeding is on the increase, but remains lowest for low-income mothers (42 percent) and for black women (37 percent).[20]

- Fewer than 20 percent of births are to black women, but they account for 40 percent of maternal deaths.[21]

• Early health deterioration has been found to contribute to poor birth outcomes among poor black women, particularly those living in low-income areas. Contrary to logic and overall medical research, for these women, giving birth after age fifteen is associated with a threefold increase in low birth weight and a fourfold increase in very low birth weight in their newborns. Although for most women it is riskier to have a baby when so young, for these women, who suffer the physical consequences of poverty, early worsening of overall health makes it riskier as they grow up.[22]

• Infant mortality among blacks declined from 18.8 per 1,000 live births in 1987 to 13.7 in 1997, still nearly double that of the total population, for which infant mortality declined from 10.1 to 7.1 over the same period. Infant mortality among migrant farm workers is 25 percent higher than the national average.[23]

• Although the prevalence of overweight among all females ages twenty to seventy-four is increasing (from 27 percent in 1980 to 37 percent in 1994), for black and Mexican-American women it remains significantly higher (52 percent and 50 percent in 1994, respectively).[24]

• Among female migrant farm workers ages fifteen to nineteen, pregnancy is the most common reason for visiting a clinic; for those ages thirty to sixty-four, the most common reasons are diabetes and hypertension; and for those sixty-five and older, 80 percent of clinic visits are for diabetes or hypertension.[25]

Underserved women in the United States need primary care. They need access to—and encouragement in seeking—cancer screenings and early prenatal care. They need counseling and education about smoking, diet, alcohol and drug abuse, heart disease risks, and risky behaviors for HIV/AIDS, as well as diabetes and hypertension management.

But simply reducing the health risks of the socioeconomically disadvantaged is not enough. A recent study at the University of Michigan shows that when health risk behaviors are accounted for, low-income groups still have a higher death risk than higher-income groups.[26] These complex health problems are often tied to social and cultural issues that make them impossible to treat effectively using traditional protocols. And, as we know, for the poor there are many obstacles to health care in addition to its cost (see Chapter Nine).

Social problems such as unemployment, lack of education, low self-esteem, domestic violence, and gangs may not be the responsibility of the health care provider, but they have an impact on health status and subsequently the utilization of health care services. Living with danger and the fear of violence, for example, creates trauma and often results in community-wide feelings of alienation, powerlessness, and hopelessness. These feelings have been linked to poor health behaviors, more doctors' visits, and significantly lower levels of preventive care.[27]

Collaboration for Success

The complexity of poverty is enough to make hospital CEOs wonder if the problem is greater than their ability to fix it. It is. And that is exactly the point. Given the magnitude of the problem, health care providers can't go it alone when developing strategies—or shouldering the cost of initiatives—to address these issues. The efforts that have demonstrated success are collaborative ones that involve universities, schools, employers, public health departments, police, parks departments, and libraries. Health is not just a provider concern; it touches the entire community.

Once you have identified your underserved populations, your next step is to identify the other stakeholders; only then you can develop your strategy. Let's look at some examples.

Lehigh Valley Hospital and Health Network has served over twenty-three hundred low-income women through its Perinatal Partnership program. The program "extends health care beyond the hospital walls by linking Lehigh Valley Hospital with community resources," according to Joan Linnander, program director. "The program is the first of its kind in Pennsylvania to draw from private funding sources, demonstrating how the two sectors can work together to improve the delivery of health and social services to the low-income population." Much of the program's success comes from breaking down language and transportation barriers through the use of bilingual community outreach workers, a satellite clinic, and free van service with a bilingual driver. The result of collaboration of local schools, churches, businesses, and citizens, the program boasts significant results:

- Preterm births among low-income women dropped to 6.1 percent from 13.3 percent; low birth weight births dropped from 12 percent to 5.3 percent.

- First-trimester prenatal care rose from 57.5 percent to 70 percent (93 percent for those women who had contact with an outreach worker).
- The rate by which low-income women returned for postpartum appointments rose to 73.3 percent from 47 percent.[28]

Sometimes collaboration takes a more nontraditional approach. In Schenectady, New York, high-risk, low-income black women weren't taking advantage of breast cancer screening, so beauty salons and churches were identified as distribution points.[29] In Anchorage, Alaska, a local cab company provides discounted fares for underserved women when they travel to mammogram appointments. In the Seattle area, competing hospitals joined together with the Department of Public Health and over fifty community groups to wrestle with tough issues of domestic violence, child abuse, teen health risks, breast cancer and maternal and infant health. "We realized that hospital lines were artificial, geopolitical things," says Keith Cernak, the alliance's director. "The search for how we could have the greatest impact led us to cross those boundaries."[30]

Hood River Memorial Hospital is the only hospital in Oregon remarkable for its high percentage of residents living below the poverty level and for its high prevalence of maternal risk factors. Multiple agencies (La Familia Sana, La Clinica del Carino, Next Door, Inc., and others) do what they can to alleviate these problems, but providers were isolated from each other and struggling to educate as well as treat their patients. The hospital worked with the Oregon Health Sciences University Library to implement a program allowing librarians to train agencies and providers to use the Internet as a source for patient education materials. Computer equipment and Internet access were provided through grant funding. Collateral and educational materials were adapted to lower reading levels, when necessary, or read to groups of those unable to read.[31]

St. Mary's Hospital of Rochester, New York, works with area volunteers to reduce the city's high rate of teen pregnancy, infant mortality, and low birth weight through an innovative effort called Healthy Moms. Welcoming each participant with a baby shower attended by former graduates, the program provides medical care, risk reduction education, and counseling in parenting and home safety. The program's most creative innovation is the appointment of a *doula*—Greek for woman's servant—to each mom-to-be, who remains her advocate throughout her pregnancy.[32]

Using Community Health Workers

There is a real opportunity for health care leaders to learn from grass-roots programs like the Mountain Scouts in eastern Kentucky, which trains "scouts" (community health workers) to educate and encourage rural, low-income women to participate in early detection screenings for cervical and breast cancer. Project Vida in El Paso, Texas, recruits patients as volunteers and salaried community health workers to help bring services to the poor, uninsured, predominantly Hispanic community. Even in Hollywood, the Los Angeles Free Clinic Hollywood Center uses peer counselors to move troubled, vulnerable young people off the streets. In Monroe, Michigan, the Camp Health Aide program trains migrant and seasonal farm workers as health aides.[33] The success of peer programs is probably largely due to their nonthreatening nature: neighbors talk to neighbors in their own homes, in their own ways, and in their own language.

Hospital-based peer programs are new but growing because of their effectiveness in reaching the hard-to-reach. This is perhaps the best current approach for breaking down stubborn barriers to health care. Johns Hopkins University School of Medicine in Baltimore, in cooperation with Johns Hopkins Hospital, received a grant from the Robert Wood Johnson Foundation to develop a new substance abuse center that will be staffed with community health workers. "Our hospital has truly come to understand the importance of its relationship to the community," says Betsy McCaw, who runs the hospital's drug treatment programs. "For a long time, hospitals have tried to isolate themselves, and Hopkins is no exception, but now we're coming around to the fact that hospitals' true strengths lie in their ability to work with and help the community—not to be the castle on the hill. We're finding CHWs are a good way of helping us do that."[34]

A strong case for the use of community health workers is made by an Austin, Texas, study in which 923 Mexican-American women were interviewed about their knowledge and attitudes about Pap smear and mammogram screening practices. According to the findings, women who are more knowledgeable are more likely to have had a recent screening. Women with only Medicare or Medicaid know far less than uninsured women. Women who do not speak English well are more likely to remain ignorant of critical cancer signs and symptoms, risk factors, and screening guidelines. Those with a fatalistic attitude are less likely to have ever had a Pap smear. The study authors conclude that low screening participation among Mexican-American women may be due to their limited awareness and language barriers, which highlights the need for interventions consistent with Mexican-American beliefs.[35]

A study at Denver General Hospital found the most important reasons for not seeking early prenatal care among low-income black, Hispanic, and white women are attitudinal in nature (47 percent), followed by financial (26 percent). The study concludes that cultural variations should be considered in developing programs intended to improve prenatal care.[36]

In addition to using peer outreach programs to overcome cultural barriers, the use of certified nurse midwives (CNMs) is becoming more popular. For many cultures, including American Indian and Hispanic, the use of midwives is centuries old, more acceptable, and more comfortable. Multiple studies document similar or better outcomes with the use of CNMs for low-income women.[37]

The mission of St. Mary's Health Network emphasizes the sanctity of life from the moment of conception and charity for those in need. But the network was struggling to bring care to those who needed it most. In the poor neighborhood of southeast Reno, infant mortality, low birth weight, and low child immunization rates were the priority issues. The decision was made to establish the Midwife and Well-Child Program and operate it in a neighborhood health center. In its first year, the program delivered 239 babies and referred sixty high-risk patients to the hospital. The average birth weight was seven pounds, one ounce. Early prenatal care and immunization rates increased. One new mother described her experience: "The best thing about St. Mary's Midwife Program was the way I was treated. From day one, everyone from the receptionists to the nurses were kind, gentle, trustworthy, and loving."[38]

A nationwide program that spans cultures to reach teenagers all across America is Crittenton Services of Nashville, founded in the 1880s originally as a chain of mission homes for unwed mothers. Today the program's mission is to prevent first and repeat teen pregnancies and teach parenting skills to pregnant teens. It does this with the help of local schools, hospitals, and volunteers, including teens who teach their peers about abstinence and encourage educational goals. Seventy-five percent of the three thousand students participating indicated a renewed commitment to abstinence or a reduction in risky behaviors; 90 percent of students enrolled in the pregnant and parenting teens program graduated from high school in 1997 (the national rate is 50 percent), and only 3.5 percent of parenting clients experienced a repeat pregnancy, compared to 50 percent nationwide.[39]

Out in the Country

In many of America's isolated mountain, prairie, backwoods, or desert regions, one might drive for hours before finding a hospital or even a doctor's office. To tackle this problem, Congress passed the Rural Clinics Act of 1977. According to the Health Care Finance Administration's 1997 count, there are now 3,270 rural health clinics (RHCs) in the United States. This represents a significant increase from 1992, when there were only 947. This growth is largely due to financial incentives designed to stimulate the establishment of more clinics. Today, however, the government is concerned that the expansion may be out of control: "While increases in the number of RHCs may improve access to health care in certain geographic areas, the RHCs are also locating in areas where Medicare and Medicaid beneficiaries already have adequate access to primary care services."[40] HCFA is pursuing plans to moderate this trend by reevaluating the shortage area designation, better identifying areas with primary care access problems, and revising the RHC payment methodology.

In some rural areas, medical and agricultural schools and universities have taken a leadership role in bringing health care to the underserved. For example, the North Carolina student rural health coalition is an organization of health professionals and volunteers who run free clinics and other interventions aimed at redressing the third world health conditions found in rural North Carolina.[41] A program developed by Texas A&M works to improve health in rural communities in three ways: increasing the number of community groups focusing on health issues, implementing a health volunteer program, and providing additional health education and activities in rural communities.[42] The University of California has targeted migrant health centers with a program designed to help them treat health problems resulting from exposure to environmental factors in the agricultural workplace, such as dusts, pesticides, and fertilizers.[43]

The University of Virginia (UVA) is wrestling with the problem of recruiting nurses to practice in underserved rural areas. Beginning with the theory that students will stay and work in their home community if they are allowed to learn there, UVA implemented a "distance learning" program funded by a Health Resources Services Administration grant. It brings nursing courses to remote areas via two-way real-time interactive compressed video, along with telephone and e-mail connections. On-site clinical coordinators, experienced nurses who work in those environments and regular visits from UVA staff, support students with a human connection. The results? Sixty to seventy percent of graduates accept positions in underserved communities. "I was overwhelmed by the appreciation shown, especially in the far southwest Virginia community. It has been a collaborative, grassroots effort with participation from all sides," said Julie Novak, director of the program.[44]

These examples begin to reveal the many ways health care providers have been joining with other stakeholders to lessen the disparity in the services offered to various population segments. Such efforts must be well supported to counterbalance a common problem in the rural health care system: physician retention. In a monograph for the National Association of Community Health Centers, Stephen D. Wilhide, president and CEO of Southern Ohio Health Services Network, points out several important factors that influence retention:[45]

- Good recruitment
- Relationship strengthening
- Continuous communication
- Recognition of efforts
- Professional autonomy
- Competitive salaries
- Collaboration in establishing productivity standards
- Authority to hire and supervise clinical staff
- Participation in managed care decisions

DELIVERING EFFECTIVE HEALTH CARE SERVICES

One challenge for health care executives is to review policies to identify creative ways of altering the health care climate in which they operate. For example, important strategies to increase access and combat rising costs for the underserved include establishing incentives for minorities to enter the medical profession,[46] for physicians to practice primary care,[47] and for physicians, physician assistants, and nurses to practice in underserved areas.[48]

To make any strategy feasible, collaboration is the key. Mobilizing resources and initiating a grassroots effort is important not only because a program has a better chance of engaging a community if it is developed and operated by the community but also because there are many other primary stakeholders in community health. By bringing together leaders from business, health care, government, and the community, there is an opportunity to create a map of resources to better identify the community's needs, strengths, and barriers. The need for funding becomes a community issue rather than simply a provider issue. Most importantly, collaboration creates an environment where the goals, outcomes, and risks are shared by all stakeholders.

Help for funding may occur at the national level. The Health Resources Services Administration (www.hrsa.gov), a division of the Health and Human Resources Department (www.hhs.gov), designates medically underserved populations and medically underserved areas, along with health professional shortage areas. The agency's goal is to assure equitable access to quality health care services for underserved and vulnerable populations through partnerships with state and local governments and community-based public and private sector organizations. State-specific data and grant information is available through these agencies and their Web sites.

Framework for the Planning Process

As with most complex enterprises, careful planning is everything when it comes to developing a strategy for health services delivery to underserved populations. The following steps illustrate the process that might be used to develop one for underserved women.

COMMUNITY ANALYSIS: ASSET MAPPING During this phase, it's important to compile a profile of the community using primary and secondary research. This involves defining the market area: what are its boundaries, population and demographics, industries, social structure, leadership, environmental conditions, and climate? What is the current health status, as reflected in health department vital statistics (for example, teen pregnancy rates, infant mortality, suicide attempts, birth weights, and mortality rates from all causes)? What are the lifestyle and health behavior patterns? What does an overview of health insurance coverage indicate? What possible competitors are there? What is the history of collaboration in the community? What other providers, higher education and other school systems, social service organizations, nonprofits, women's community groups, medical staff and community, government, business and business organizations might become community partners? What are the community's capacities and assets, from human resources and dollars to readiness to accept the project? Are there barriers to implementation? The answers to these questions are the basis for an asset map of community resources.

INSTITUTIONAL ANALYSIS   This step can include a SWOT analysis (strengths, weaknesses, opportunities, and threats) of your organization; a historical perspective of your organization (including operational, marketing, product and service offerings, and financial overviews); a competitive overview; resource identification (including staffing, volunteers, capital improvement, cash on hand, potential, board, and the like); and review of strategic plans and initiatives and managed care participation.

PROGRAM INITIATION: RESOURCES LEVERAGING   This step involves developing strategies and tactics, timelines, and budgets. It requires recruiting citizens for membership on task forces and work groups and establishing a core planning group, including a project coordinator and champions. It requires people to choose an organizational structure; mission, goals, and expected measures of success; and roles, responsibilities, strategies, and methods. It's also important to identify measures to track for evaluation; collect baseline data; and design evaluation methodology. An aggressive communications and public relations strategy must be developed and put in place. A community leadership team must be convened, with emphasis on influential women. Training and recognition for volunteers, participants, and staff must be provided. Collaborative opportunities should be identified in which other partners contribute resources and take responsibility for shared goals and shared outcomes. Outside funding sources (government and foundation grants, in-kind contributions, individual contributors, partner funding) should be identified.

IMPLEMENTATION AND OPERATION: BECOMING VIABLE   The organization should function as a small business unit with strict measures of accountability, commit to a proactive reporting format, track and measure outcomes (performance measures), and share these publicly.

DISSEMINATION AND REASSESSMENT   The effectiveness of programs must be measured continuously. Evaluation should be used to drive planning of programs, funding, and management, and results should be summarized and disseminated to the community at large. Semi-annual reporting to community leaders and decision makers, policy-makers, patients, partners, and others should emphasize results and progress. The current environment should be assessed on an ongoing basis (updating the asset map) to determine program need and effectiveness, identify and remove barriers, and identify successes and build on them.

LONGEVITY: EARNING THE RIGHT TO CONTINUE TO SERVE   To serve over the long term, it's important to pool community resources—manpower, capital, and in-kind services. In addition, pursue augmentative funding sources (such as grants) and manage the budget. Finally, your keep eyes and ears open to identify what is not working and change it.

A Word About Evaluation

One of the most important agenda items to tackle in planning is perhaps the most often neglected: evaluation. Solid measures of positive outcomes can help you secure ongoing funding. But if you wait to think about evaluation until the annual report is due, it is too late. For effective measurement and evaluation, start early. This means building clearly quantifiable goals into the initial strategy. Then, with those goals in mind, do the following:

- Gather all available baseline data related to goals. For example, capture the health status, health behaviors, utilization patterns, and health outcomes of the targeted population regarding the specific services or health issues to be addressed, as well as the cost of relevant care. Survey or interview a representative sample regarding their perceptions of and attitudes about the quality and accessibility of health care services.
- Make it a part of every encounter to gather the data needed to track the program's impact on all the identified measures.

• Delegate analysis of the collected data to an objective third party with expertise in community health and data analysis.

SUMMARY

Management may not see underserved women as a source of revenue. But given women's role as gatekeeper for family health and the importance that primary and preventative care have on efficient and cost-effective utilization, creating a strategy for serving this audience may, in fact, be critical to the bottom line. Indeed, serving the now underserved woman may soon need to be integrated with other critical financial and strategic objectives of providers if they want to succeed in the future.

Following the dollar—not necessarily in terms of revenue today but in terms of possible lost revenue later—delivers us to the obvious conclusion. Five variables are certain:

• Demographic projections indicate that women will continue to be in the majority of the underserved.

• The underserved woman is not that different from her peer whose health care is covered by a generous self-insured employer: both usually make the health care decisions for their families.

• Inappropriate utilization of health care services by any population served in a managed care environment will cost the health care provider money.

• With decreasing Medicaid and Medicare reimbursement, providers will continue to be asked to do more for less.

• Within this framework, prevention and health management strategies become good business objectives.

With health care resources becoming tighter and demand for services increasing, it makes good business sense to develop aggressive strategies to address the needs of underserved populations. From an operational perspective, the following first steps can be a pragmatic response to the issue:

• Analyze and streamline patient flow procedures.

- Expand primary care services and create smoother linkages between community service agencies and specialty care.

- Commit to a multidisciplinary approach. Focus on health promotion activities, female inpatient services, and pre- and perinatal care.

- Recognize the unique needs of specific population groups: underserved older women, various cultures, adolescents.

- Become the central hub for disseminating health information throughout your community, such as in churches, schools, community centers, grocery stores, and beauty salons.

- Use refined tools to measure patient satisfaction.

- Track access and utilization patterns for the demographic groups in the underserved population.

- Pool data with others across the community to analyze what is working and what is not.

These are important steps, for addressing the needs of underserved women and their families will remain a critical strategic issue for health care providers positioning for viability long into the new millennium.

Notes

1. Fisher, M. J. "Insurers Caution Congress on Health Reform." *National Underwriter Property and Casualty-Risk Benefits Management,* Jan. 11, 1999, *103*(2), 6.
2. Iglehart, J. K. "The American Health Care System: Expenditures." *New England Journal of Medicine,* 1999, *340*(1), 27.
3. "C. Everett Koop Community Health Awards." [http//healthproject .stanford.edu/koop/community/criteria.html]; Russell, L. B. "Prevention and Medicare Costs." *New England Journal of Medicine,* 1998, *339*(16); "Healthy Cities." [http://www.healthycities.org]; Gale, B. J. "Faculty Practice as Partnership with a Community Coalition." *Journal of Professional Nursing,* 1998, *14*(5), 267–271; Centers for Disease Control and Prevention. "Pregnant Women, Infants and the Cost Savings of Smoking Cessation." Washington, D.C.: Centers for Disease Control and Prevention, 1997; Banks, D. A., Paterson, M., and Wendel, J. "Uncompensated Hospital Care: Charitable Mission or Profitable Business Decision?" *Health Economics,* 1997, *6*(2), 133–143.

4. Pelletier, K. "A Review and Analysis of the Health and Cost-Effective Outcome Studies of Comprehensive Health Promotion and Disease Prevention Programs at the Worksite." *American Journal of Health Promotion,* 1996, *10*(5), 380–388; Ziegler, J. "America's Healthiest Companies." *Business and Health,* Dec. 1998, pp. 29–31; Lukes, E. "Medical Surveillance Program Evaluation: Successful Program." *Journal of the American Association of Occupational Health Nursing,* 1998, *46*(12), 574–580; Gray, C. "Wellness Program Payback." *Modern Healthcare,* 1996, *14:26*(42), 72–78.

5. Gavin, N. I., and others. "The Use of EPSDT and Other Health Care Services by Children Enrolled in Medicaid: The Impact of OBRA '89." *Milbank Quarterly,* 1998, *2,* 207–250.

6. Carpenter, M. B., and Kavanagh, L. D. "Outreach and State Children's Health Insurance Program: Helping States Enroll Children and Assure Access to Care." Paper presented at the National Center for Education in Maternal and Child Health at Georgetown University, Washington D.C., Dec. 1997.

7. Summer, L., Carpenter, M. B., and Kavanagh, L. D. *Successful Outreach Strategies: Ten Programs That Link Children to Health Services.* Washington, D.C.: Health Resources Administration, U.S. Department of Health and Human Services, 1999.

8. Summary of "Improved Maternal and Children's Health Coverage Act of 1999," bill to be introduced into the House of Representatives by Reps. Diana DeGette (D-Colo.) and Connie Morella (R-Md.).

9. Adams, K., Oliver, R., Custer, W., and Ketsche, P. "An Overview of Health Reform, Their Effects and Relationship to the Medicaid Program." Unpublished manuscript. Emory University Rollins School of Public Health and Georgia State University Center for Risk Management and Insurance Research; Simpson, L., Korenbrot, C., and Green, J. "Outcomes of Enhanced Prenatal Services for Medicaid-Eligible Women in Public and Private Settings." *Public Health Reports,* 1997, *112*(2), 122–132; Salganicoff, A. "Medicaid and Managed Care: Implications for Low-Income Women." *Journal of the American Medical Women's Association,* 1997, *52*(2), 78–80.

10. General Accounting Office. *Arizona Medicaid: Competition Among Managed Care Plans Lowers Program Costs.* Washington, D.C.: General Accounting Office, 1995.

11. Bennefield, R. L. *Current Population Reports: Consumer Income; Health Insurance Coverage, 1997.* Washington, D.C.: U.S. Department of Commerce, Economics and Statistics Administration, 1998, pp. 60–202.

12. National Coalition for the Homeless, Feb. 1999. [http://nch.ari.net].

13. Salit, S. A., and others. "Hospitalization Costs Associated with Homelessness in New York City." *New England Journal of Medicine,* 1999, *338*(24), 132–133.

14. Migrant Health Program. [http://www.bphc.hrsa.dhhs.gov/mhc/MIGRANT.html]; National Center for Farmworker Health. [http://www.ncfh.org].

15. "Women's Health in the States: Current Issues and Trends." [http://www.jiwh.org/current/htm].

16. Handler, A., Raube, K., Kelley, M. A., and Giachello, A. "Women's Satisfaction with Prenatal Care Settings: A Focus Group Study." *Birth,* 1996, *23*(1), 31–37.

17. Handler, A., Rosenberg, D., Raube, K., and Kelley, M. A. "Health Care Characteristics Associated with Women's Satisfaction with Prenatal Care." *Medical Care,* 1998, *36*(5), 679–694.

18. Harper, M. "The Health of Minority Women." Paper presented at the History and Future of Women's Health conference, Public Health Service Office on Women's Health, June 1998.

19. Harper, "The Health of Minority Women."

20. Harper, "The Health of Minority Women."

21. Harper, "The Health of Minority Women."

22. U.S. Department of Health and Human Services. *Healthy People 2000 Progress Review: Women's Health.* Washington, D.C.: U.S. Government Printing Office, 1998.

23. U.S. Department of Health and Human Services, *Healthy People 2000 Progress Review: Women's Health.*

24. U.S. *Department of Health and Human Services. Healthy People 2000 Progress Review: Black Americans.* Washington, D.C.: U.S. Government Printing Office, 1998.

25. Geronimus, A. T. "Black/White Differences in the Relationship of Maternal Age to Birthweight: A Population-Based Test of the Weathering Hypothesis." *Social Science and Medicine,* 1996, *42*(4), 589–597.

26. U.S. Department of Health and Human Services. *Healthy People 2000 Progress Review: Hispanic Americans.* Washington, D.C.: U.S. Government Printing Office, 1997.

27. National Center for Farmworker Health. [http://www.ncfh.org].

28. U.S. Department of Health and Human Services, *Healthy People 2000 Progress Review: Women's Health.*

29. U.S. Department of Health and Human Services, *Healthy People 2000 Progress Review: Women's Health.*

30. Lantz, P. M., and others. "Socioeconomic Factors, Health Behaviors, and Mortality: Results from a Nationally Representative Prospective Study of U.S. Adults." *Journal of the American Medical Association*, 1998, *279*(21), 1703–1708.

31. Phillips, K. S. "The Ecology of Urban Violence: Its Relationship to Health Promotion Behaviors in Low-Income Black and Latino Communities." *American Journal of Health Promotion*, 1996, *10*(2), 308–315.

32. "Perinatal Partnership Shows Strong Results for Low-Income Women, Newborns in the Lehigh Valley." [http://www.lvhhn.org/aboutus /press_releases/9605/960502a.html].

33. "Perinatal Partnership."

34. Centers for Disease Control and Prevention. "Surprising Barriers Prevent Women from Seeking Breast Cancer Screening." Bethesda, Md.: National Center for Health Statistics, 1998.

35. Speer, T. "Bridges Make Good Neighbors." *Hospitals & Health Networks*, Jan. 1998, pp. 55–56.

36. "Oregon Community Health Outreach Project." [http://www.nnlm.nlm.nih.gov/pnr/specproj/orecom.html].

37. Larson, L., and Lumsdon, K. "Their Turf, Their Terms." *Hospitals & Health Networks*, Sept. 1996, pp. 48–50.

38. U.S. Department of Health and Human Services. "Small Investments in Health Care Yield Big Payoffs for Poor, Uninsured and Underserved." Washington, D.C.: U.S. Government Printing Office, 1996.

39. Skinner, C. S., and others. "Learn, Share and Live: Breast Cancer Education for Older, Urban Minority Women." *Health Education and Behavior*, 1998, *25*(1), 60–78.

40. Sherer, J. "Neighbor to Neighbor: Community Health Workers Educate Their Own." *Hospitals & Health Networks*, Oct. 1994, pp. 52–56.

41. Suarez, L., Roche, R. A., Nichols, D., and Simpson, D. M. "Knowledge, Behavior, and Fears Concerning Breast and Cervical Cancer Among Older Low-Income Mexican-American Women." *American Journal of Preventive Medicine*, 1997, *13*(2), 137–142.

42. Meikle, S. F., and others. "Women's Reasons for Not Seeking Prenatal Care: Racial and Ethnic Factors." *Birth*, 1995, *22*(2), 81–86.

43. Blanchette, H. "Comparison of Obstetric Outcome of a Primary-Care Access Clinic Staffed by Certified Nurse-Midwives and a Private Practice Group of Obstetricians in the Same Community." *American Journal of Obstetrics and Gynecology*, 1995, *172*(6), 184–188; Fischler, N. R., and Harvey, S. M. "Setting and Provider of Prenatal Care: Association with

Pregnancy Outcomes Among Low-Income Women." *Health Care for Women International,* 1995, *16*(4), 309–321; Welch, K. "Women's Health and Low-Income Housing." *Journal of Midwifery,* 1997, *42*(6), 521–526.

44. "The Spirit of Innovation Awards." [http://www.mmm.com/market /healthcare/interhealth/soi/96SOIDP57.html].

45. Crittenton Services of Nashville, Tenn. [http://www.birdsnbees.org].

46. Statement of Kathleen A. Buto, associate administrator for policy, Health Care Financing Administration, on "rural health clinics" before the House Committee on Government Reform and Oversight, Subcommittee on Human Resources and Intergovernmental Relations, Feb. 13, 1997. [http://www.hcfa.gov/testimony/rural.htm].

47. "NC Student Rural Health Coalition, Duke Med Chapter." [http://www.duke.edu/web/ncsrhc-dumc/mission.htm].

48. "Health Education Rural Outreach Program." Texas A&M University. [http://fcs.tamu.edu/health/hero.htm].

CHAPTER ELEVEN

Getting the Most from Each Marketing Dollar

Genie James

B efore addressing how to get the most for every marketing dollar spent promoting a women's health initiative, it is essential to first define what marketing really means. Most executives realize that the term can embrace communication, advertising, outreach, and goodwill. Unfortunately, very few demonstrate an active understanding of the fact that honest-to-goodness marketing is the vehicle by which strategic direction becomes operational. Marketing is an umbrella term that includes the following:

- Mass-marketing and multiple-media campaigns
- Community education and outreach
- Physician and medical staff relations
- Patient satisfaction monitoring
- Health fairs
- Wellness events
- Managed care promotions
- Trustee relations

In today's health care industry, providers are operating in a highly competitive and resource constrained environment. A marketing initiative should be the means by which various stakeholders and customer groups are made aware of and then sold an idea. If you are committed to selling a women's health strategy, you need to commit your energies to a matrix selling process which requires tailoring your message to multiple audiences. Senior administrators, physician champions, trustee leaders, and key managed care payors are foremost among those that you want to understand how your proposed strategy will benefit them.

ESTABLISHING SYSTEMS FOR ACCOUNTABILITY AND PERFORMANCE MEASURES

For a women's health focus to be taken seriously from the very beginning, it is essential to establish a system of accountability that can track a return on any financial investment. It is also essential to assign responsibility and to identify who will take the lead in communicating outcomes to the stakeholders. Doing the "right thing" requires earning the right to do so; accountability is essential.

How do you go about convincing stakeholders? First, conduct enough market intelligence to ensure that you are fully aware of each individual's unique motivators. Then tailor your message accordingly. For instance, a physician leader may have greatest interest when you describe the potential new patients that a program could bring through the doors. Your CEO may be more motivated by discussions of market share and revenue. A trustee whose mother or sister is a breast cancer survivor may have a passion for education and early intervention programs. All these people are primary customers that must be sold on an idea before it can be implemented.

Understanding what motivates your audience sounds basic but it is the most frequently bungled step. At a 1998 workshop for marketing directors working in hospitals managed by Quorum Health Resources, Inc., participants were asked to introduce themselves and to describe all the functions—besides marketing—for which they were responsible. They wore a variety of hats, as do most department managers today. Marketing responsibilities were most often grouped with community outreach activities; in several organizations, marketing was grouped with business development or managed care functions. One person even indicated that he was responsible for physical plant maintenance. But when asked how many of them were considered part of a senior management team, very few raised their hands.

SELLING WOMEN'S HEALTH WITHIN THE ORGANIZATION

The same group was presented with several puzzle pieces with one of the following headings inscribed on each: mission/vision, ambulatory facilities, changes in reimbursement, physician partnerships, managed care strategy, community service, network affiliations, and marketing. Asked to pretend that they were the CEO of the hospital in which they worked and to indicate which two their CEO would pick up, no one picked up the marketing piece. Herein lies a basic problem.

The first challenge for anyone passionate about a women's health strategy is to internally sell its importance and potential impact. Marketing women's health to senior-level decision makers requires much more than image building. It requires a real understanding of what your CEO and hospital board regard as the strategic priorities for your organization. Your objectives associated with women's health should then be positioned in such a way to be viewed as complementary or supportive of these very same initiatives. See Table 11.1.

Suppose that the most critical issue that your organization faces is outmigration and a subsequent increase in market share. Because women have been documented as the primary health care decision makers for their families, a women's health initiative can be positioned internally as one means to achieve an increase in patient flow and hospital revenue. Similarly, if physician partnerships are where your organization is vesting time and money, the opportunity to capture new patients and upstream referrals should be highlighted.

Although in today's tumultuous reimbursement environment mission and vision too often get short shift, there are still organizations who demonstrate an authenticity of purpose that is in alignment with their mission statement. This is particularly true if the organization is not-for-profit because the need to protect a tax exempt status is a very real business issue. If this is the case for your hospital or health system, then you have a real opportunity to position your women's health strategy simply by the very fact that any outreach activities will affect the underserved female consumers. If you are savvy in matching up your initiatives with the need to substantiate and measure your orga-

Cultural Realities	Strategic Objectives	Tactical Activities
Clear focus on customer satisfaction	Analysis of market research, quantitative and qualitative	Internal communications External communications
Customer service	Assessment of competitive	Planning and execution
Innovation and leadership	positioning: opportunities and threats	Public relations Advertising
Internal champions positioned across the continuum	Formulation of a strategy Transference of strategic information Implementation of program/product development Government relations/ fit with policy	Pricing Sales Tracking Feedback loops

Table 11.1. Key Success Factors for Marketing Strategies.
Source: Adapted from *Health Marketing Quarterly*, 1997, vol. 15.

nization's commitment to serving its community, then you will not only enhance the visibility of your programs but also garner the buy-in of your trustees, which can facilitate their willingness to support other initiatives you may put on the table.

MARKETING MAKES ITS MARK

Here are examples that demonstrate both creativity and a commitment to using marketing to get results. First is a hospital that differentiated itself within a very competitive marketplace where everyone had a version of a breast cancer awareness program. Second is a nationwide partnership of health care organizations, leading in the area of women's health.

Small-Scale Approach to Prevention

Florida Hospital in Orlando, an 1,111-bed facility, generated a large community response by promoting mammography with a tiny direct mail piece—a 21/2-by-1-inch box containing a minuscule booklet, a packet of wildflower seeds, and a coupon for a discounted mammogram. The box and booklet are decorated with striking watercolor paintings and urge women to "Celebrate Life." The booklet notes that a flower seed is about the size of a breast cancer that can be detected by mammograms. As Karla Cole, advertising manager for Florida Hospital who developed the campaign, says, "We wanted a very positive approach—emphasizing prevention rather than negative scare tactics." The hospital mailed twenty thousand flower boxes to its community in the spring of 1990 and twenty thousand that fall. Nearly five hundred women responded by redeeming the coupon for a discounted mammogram. The campaign cost $40,000—and generated an estimated $727,000 in additional patient visits. Business people may celebrate such a significant return on investment; most importantly, the piece is saving lives.[1]

Strategic Alliance and Partnership

The Spirit of Women partnership leverages efforts on a community level with access to the resources of national corporate sponsorship.[2] Spirit of Women is unique in its goal of combining local women's health programming with major corporate marketing efforts. This mission is attained through the following goals:

- To strengthen the strategic position of the member as the regional leader of health services for women through the use of national sponsors, spokespeople, and the affiliation of other recognized health facilities.

- To gather national resources for use in local applications. These applications will be directed by the member in a unique national partnership.

- To heighten the existing ability of participants to impact the primary health care decision makers (women) who also make health plan choices in a managed care environment.

- To provide a national resource of funding specifically for women's health issues through the creation of a Spirit of Women Foundation.

- To provide a national forum where members interact in the development and formation of responses to the evolving health needs of women in markets across the United States.

Spirit of Women began as a local initiative of Lehigh Valley Hospital and Health Network in Allentown, Pennsylvania, pioneered by women's health director Marie Shaw. As the local leader in women's health, Lehigh Valley Hospital was focused on offering the best in women's health education to coincide with the excellent clinical care it provided. An annual women's health forum continued to expand to include over 750 women in a two-day conference format.

The Spirit of Women network is made up of health care organizations, corporate sponsors, and the general partners. *Prevention,* the nation's twelfth-largest magazine and the most widely circulated health and wellness magazine, is an integral partner in this initiative. Not only is *Prevention* preeminent in the health publications arena, it also has strong national sponsor connections to lend to this program.

Lehigh Valley Hospital came to Medimetrix Unison Marketing, located in Englewood, Colorado, to expand partnership and bring it to a national level. Together they have initiated this effort in close to two dozen hospitals and health systems.

Program benefits to be evaluated by hospitals and health systems considering joining the Spirit of Women Health Network include the following:

- Positions the hospital or health system as a major player in women's issues through association with national sponsors, national spokespersons, and partnership with market leaders in women's health.

- Brings major sponsors and more affordable national spokeswomen to regional events. This creates marketing and public relations opportunities beyond what individuals could do as a single effort.

- Extends credibility through editorial support in *Prevention* magazine.

- Increases ability to solicit local sponsors and partners for regional women's events by providing increased media and national sponsorship.

- Provides public relations benefits of regional and national Spirit of Women Awards.

- Allows use of the Spirit of Women logo in all company and brand advertising, promotion, and publicity not directly associated with the program for duration of contract.

- Offers access to additional women's programming marketing services at preferred rates from additional national companies.

- Provides a high-value marketing campaign at a fraction of the cost to produce TV, print, radio, and collaterals.

Spirit of Women has gotten off to a great start. As Tanya Ozor, director of marketing communications and Womancare International at Magee Women's Hospital in Pittsburgh, says, "The collaborative effort and sharing of resources offers some interesting benefits to the member health care organizations. In addition to bringing women together, this program gives our physicians who care for women the opportunity to connect with colleagues across the country. In the long run, this will provide added benefit to the women they care for." It will be interesting to track the momentum of this program over the next few years. The big question remains: Will providers feel that they realize a substantial return on investment?

Outsourcing Marketing

In the fall of 1998, a customer forum sponsored by Aegis Marketing in Nashville, Tennessee, was attended by more than forty representatives of its hospital and health system customers. Many of the hospital representatives were not marketing directors but were CEOs, CFOs, or senior vice presidents charged with business development and managed care responsibilities. They were choosing to partner with Aegis because they viewed marketing as a critical component of their local market strategy and because they wanted to work with an expert partner in leveraging a relationship with local employers. One of the most powerful strategic moves possible is that of making alliances between providers and targeted employers. Doing business with employers in the community means directly influencing the purchasing decisions of insured consumers where they work, not where they live.

Although Aegis's products and services are not designed specifically for the female employee, anecdotal reports indicated that the employers recognized that—whatever marketing materials were used—it would be the women in the workplace who would determine its success. So far, the evidence indicates that Aegis is definitely doing something right. Its program includes five basic components:[3]

1. The Health Information Center (HIC) is a top-quality, wall-mounted display designed to educate employees on pertinent health issues and promote the hospital in the workplace. Mea-

suring thirty-five by forty-two inches, the HIC is strategically placed in high-traffic locations inside each business. It includes the following.

Body-mind display: a professional poster-publication that offers employees easy-to-read articles on a variety of health topics

Personal health guides: a series of four take-away cards containing information on healthy living and personal well-being

Hospital advertisement: an opportunity for the hospital to present a different marketing message each month

2. The Consumer Acquisition and Profiling System (CAPS) software organizes demographic and health history information collected from employees on reply cards during on-site visits. This data is then used to develop a health profile of each company from which a hospital can sell services—based on the documented need of each employer. The data also serves as the basis for revenue-generating database marketing campaigns.

3. MedExpress Paks, mailed monthly, provide employers with relevant information about the health and wellness events sponsored by the hospital.

4. On-Site Wellness Events are offered to employers in the hospital's market on a monthly basis; Aegis helps the hospital refocus events that are already provided—cholesterol screenings, flu shots, stress management seminars, and the like—directly on employers. These on-site events maximize the effectiveness of the Aegis program and promote the hospital in the business community.

5. The Market Specialist, a trained Aegis employee, manages all of these activities on behalf of the hospital and serves as the liaison with businesses in your market, keeping your name in front of employers and becoming your "pulse on the marketplace."

EXTENDING AN INVITATION
TO WOMEN IN THE COMMUNITY

The Nashville YWCA and Saint Thomas Health Services collaborated to sponsor a women's health event that was a joint celebration of their respective one hundred years of service in Nashville and surrounding areas. The event, entitled "The Balancing Act," was a success. Health screenings began at 7:00 A.M., followed by a healthy breakfast in the dining room. After brief introductions, the keynote speaker, Deborah Norville, addressed the guests with anecdotes from her life. Afterward, there were breakout sessions covering topics important to women's health such as hormone replacement therapy, cardiovascular disease, stress reduction, senior care, alternative health remedies, and skin care. The participants could choose to attend two of these sessions. The event concluded at 11:30 A.M.

The women who attended were younger than anticipated, with most falling between thirty-five and forty-four years of age. An overwhelming majority were professionals, as expected. Almost everyone heard of the event by receiving an invitation, not through advertising. The attendees reported that they appreciated the manner in which the whole program was packaged. "When I opened my invitation, it looked just like a page from my calendar," one woman exclaimed. "It even had a yellow sticky note saying "Don't forget to take time for yourself."" Another reported, "The topics were pertinent and the keynote speaker got my attention. The morning was a great investment of my time and it made me think a little differently of both sponsoring organizations."[4]

SUMMARY

Today's marketing efforts must blend cultural realities, strategic objectives, and tactical activities. This is particularly true when marketing a women's health program because there is a danger that women's health will be subjugated to other programs associated with more immediate revenue such as cardiology or orthopedics. This chapter looked at several examples in which creativity was combined with strategic thinking to engender positive and meaningful outcomes.

In positioning your women's health program for success, remember that you do not have to do it alone. Involve stakeholders and key decision makers across your organization. Cultivate those trustees who can be your champions. Look beyond your own organization for the resources you will need to move forward to accomplish your goals.

Notes

1. Goldman, E. F. "Wellness Efforts: Hospitals Boost Education, Awareness." *American Hospital,* Apr. 20, 1992, p. 4.

2. For more information on joining the Spirit of Women Network, contact Leigh Adamson at Medimetrix Unison Marketing, 6312 South Fiddler's Green Cir., Suite 500N, Englewood, CO 80111; phone: (303) 779-3004.
3. Aegis Employer Integrated Network Program. *Helping Providers Do Business with Business.* Aegis, 1 Burton Hills Blvd., Suite 200, Nashville, TN 37215; phone: (615) 665-4200 or (800) 883-0090.
4. Perry, L. *Event Evaluation.* St. Thomas Health Services, St. Thomas Hospital, 4220 Harding Rd., Box 380, Nashville, TN 37202; phone (615) 222-2111.

PART THREE

The Hands Touching the Patients

Models for Care

This section explores models currently in use and being developed to serve the women's health care market. In Chapter Twelve, Jeffrey Persson explains the joint-equity model for physician integration, enabling providers to compare their services to it. In Chapter Thirteen, Cathy Hoot details the strengths and weaknesses of the nurse practitioner model, which is on the rise.

In Chapter Fourteen, Holly Owens describes employer strategies for serving the market and discusses whether it is best to make, rent, or buy health services for an appropriate return on investment. Jaynelle Stichler, the author of Chapter Eight, is a nationally recognized expert in women's health and health facility planning and design and a driving force behind the design and development of one of the largest women's hospitals in the United States. Thus she is well qualified to have written Chapter Fifteen, which discusses how best to create healing environments for women.

In Chapter Sixteen, Genie James and Ann Boeke discuss how to plan women's health initiatives and review case studies of three successful initiatives. Chapter Seventeen, by Kim Weiss, discusses the past, present, and future of Medicare. A topic of increasing importance to providers, Medicare is especially relevant given the aging of the population and women's dominance in that population. Chapter Eighteen explains that there is hope for the future of health care, especially in its turn toward relationship-centered care.

The conclusion of the book, Chapter Nineteen, again emphasizes why women consumers will be a defining point in the success of any health-care delivery system.

CHAPTER TWELVE

Physician Integration: When to Partner

Jeffrey B. Persson

> *Jeffrey B. Persson, senior manager of integration services for Horne CPA Group in Brentwood, Tennessee, was formerly a director of integration services with Quorum Health Resources, LLC. His previous posts also include appointments at KPMG Peat Marwick, Kaiser Permanente, and the University of Michigan Medical Center.*

The ability to organize physicians and develop a well-rounded provider base is key to the long-term viability of any health system. The physician mix of any network is a critical success factor. Because it is widely recognized that the female consumer opens her provider directory and looks first for her OB/GYN, many savvy health care providers are experimenting with the best way to build physician networks in order to secure market share and participate in the prepaid dollar stream. Two strategies are emerging in the marketplace: emerging specialty networks and acquiring physician practices.

For the past three years, OB/GYNs have been rushing to join physician practice management firms (PPMs), motivated by fear of reimbursement reductions, being squeezed out of managed care contracts, intense scrutiny by insurance carriers, and losing control of their practice and their role as patient advocates.

Emerging specialty networks have attempted to capitalize on these motivators and for awhile there was a mass stampede of physicians signing up with PPMs. For the OB/GYN wanting a single specialty model there were plenty of choices: to name just a few, GynCor, PrincipalCare, Women's Health Partners, MidSouth Health Alliance, Renaissance Centers for Women, Medisphere, and Women's Integrated Network, Inc. Unfortunately for those physicians who rushed pell-mell into these new deals, PPM firms have collided with reality. Running practices is a lot tougher than investors originally presumed, and making a profit in a climate of risk contracts and declining reimbursements can be nearly impossible. As a result, many PPMs have folded. Despite the ups and downs of the PPM industry, niche players will continue to enter a market and attempt to steal physician and market share. The need to lock in local physicians is a critical business issue. Be aware that "locking in" requires more than loyalty; it requires dollars.

Hospitals and health systems continue to struggle to find the right strategy for performing with physicians. They must have the right mix of the most-asked-for physicians and the most efficient and effective deliverers of hands-on care if they are to secure market share and to protect themselves against niche players. The joint equity model for physician integration offers hospital health systems an alternative with unique benefits in the local market. This chapter explores the joint equity model beginning with why to pursue physician integration, proceeding through how to determine whether the joint equity model is the recommended integration solution, and ending with how to develop the model.

PHYSICIAN INTEGRATION

The health care system is changing essentially every day. What worked in the past is not necessarily going to work tomorrow. During the 1980s many integrated delivery systems tried to build a continuum of care by purchasing physician practices. Many smaller hospitals and rural hospitals have, reluctantly, followed suit. Unfortunately, many of these acquisitions have been outright disasters. The reasons are many. These failures forced executives to seek not only what went wrong, but also what other alternatives might be out there.

Failures of Early Integration Efforts

Much has been written about the failure of early integration efforts; less has been written about why they failed and how they could have been better. In the 1980s many larger tertiary systems began to realize that to survive in capitated environments they would need a steady and reliable source of referrals to ensure that their specialists, and thus admissions, would be secure. The smart money back then was on building a primary care physician network. This was usually done through buying the key primary care physician practices in the service area, including OB/GYN practices, and employing the physicians. As it turns out there were a number of false assumptions with this strategy.

First, in order for a not-for-profit or a nonprofit to purchase a physician practice, the IRS requires that the purchase be made at fair market value. This can be accomplished by having an independent valuation firm perform the valuation.

Second, the major expense of any physician practice is the physician expense, including salaries, bonuses, and benefits. In many physician acquisitions, a valuation has an assumption about future physician compensation. The hospital, armed with its independent valuation, then negotiates with the physician, who agrees to sell, but only if he gets the same salary as before the transaction. Unfortunately many hospitals forgot that this has an impact on the valuation and agreed to compensation packages that were in excess of the assumption in the valuation and, thus, automatically set themselves up for operating losses even before operations began.

Third, independent physicians are used to working long hours for their compensation. This is accounted for in the valuation. But once the physician becomes a salaried employee, the incentive to work those long hours disappears.

Fourth, these acquisitions consume huge amounts of capital resources, mostly in cash. That's the front end. After the acquisition, the hospital must now run the physician practices. Very few hospital administrators or financial officers have this experience. They are excellent at hospital operations, but that is a different skill set. The result is that the physician practices are relegated to low priorities on the to-do lists and after a year or two, the hospital's reward for its integration efforts is a large capital expenditure that is now operating poorly and losing large sums of money annually. And as if that were not enough, the physicians and their staffs are dissatisfied with the whole situation. With all these problems leading to large losses in physician integration efforts, how should a health care system pursue integration in today's environment without draining the system of its capital resources only to show large operating losses?

Strategic Objectives

It's taught that form follows function. Unfortunately, what is often forgotten is that function follows strategy. It is strategy that determines what functions need to be performed—and thus which form is best. Before embarking on a joint equity project, be sure to know the strategic objectives. As shown in Figure 12.1, strategy is the foundation for everything.

Goals of Physician Integration

What are the goals of physician integration? This fundamental question has to be answered before everything else. It makes sense for physicians and the hospital to take time to state their individual and system goals and to put these on paper. This accomplishes two things: it ensures that everyone is aware of what the other parties want to achieve, and it can be used later in the process to ensure that each step taken moves closer to achieving these goals.

There are short-term and long-term goals. The short-term goal is always survival, for without survival the long-term goals become irrelevant. In the past, with cost-based reimbursement systems, survival was not much in doubt. However, in today's turbulent environment, changing reimbursement systems, government regulations, and so forth, survival should always be the basic goal.

The long-term goal is generally to develop a system for service delivery that has an impact on three categories: cost efficiency, access to care, and community health status. Cost efficiency is a key goal under capitation and many other reimbursement methodologies.

One of the most popular strategies has become the formation of specialty networks to contract with HMOs on a capitated carve-out basis. But setting up and operating a successful specialty network is a tough challenge, and the executives involved are faced with a myriad of financing options and structural decisions that must be made in a vacuum of historical knowledge and with a total void of experi-

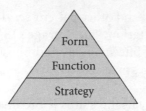

Figure 12.1.   Form Follows Function, but Function Follows Strategy.

ence. Do you include a broad range of covered services, or limit those services to a narrowly defined few? Should the network accept capitation but pay its doctors fee-for-service, or pass the capitation dollars on? How should the network and payor assign responsibility for UR and other administrative matters? How many providers will the network support?[1]

It is difficult to be a high-cost provider today and still get contracts because other providers and systems in the market can provide similar services. Given the difficulty in measuring quality of service in health care, it is imperative to be cost competitive.

Norbert Gleicher, an OB/GYN who is president and chief executive officer of GynCor, a Chicago-based physician practice management company (PPMC) specializing in reproductive medicine, says that "insurance carriers will always want to have as many general OB/GYNs as possible in their networks. Insurance company executives hate nothing more than to tell their patient population that they have to switch OB/GYN providers." OB/GYN subspecialists, however, are much more likely to be excluded from large-scale contracts unless they are part of a large, local provider organization such as an individual practice association (IPA) or a PPMC.[2]

Access to care is another key goal. Payors and patients are looking for convenience and are willing to switch providers, even at a premium, in order to get that convenience. OB/GYNs are high on the list of "most requested." Surveys reveal a heavy work load for the typical OB/GYN. The average OB/GYN work week included fifty-one hours of direct patient care activities. This included seeing patients in the office, time in the operating room or labor and delivery, making hospital rounds, seeing patients in an outpatient clinic or emergency room, seeing patients at home in nursing homes or other extended care facilities, telephone conversations with patients, consultations with other physicians, and other patient services such as laboratory test or X-ray interpretation. The average OB/GYN work week also included an additional fifteen hours of administrative activities. Physician work load becomes an essential variable in making tough structural decisions.[3]

Finally, community health status is the third goal. It is no longer acceptable to merely provide "sick care" in communities. It is important to keep communities healthy and prevent the need for care, especially expensive care like hospital care. Female consumers are highly cognizant not only of what is being done for them personally but, just as important, of how their provider of choice bears responsibility for the underserved.

Numerous specific goals are dependent on the individual circumstance of each situation. They generally fall into one of the three categories listed. However, these are what will drive the integration effort and will be the critical success factors and milestones of the integration effort.

Logic of Physician Integration

Physician integration makes good business sense; it puts all critical success factors and key initiatives into alignment. Physician integration builds a primary care base, provides strength in managed care contracting, is an innovative outpatient strategy, aligns physician and hospital incentives, and improves access for the community.

Although there are already primary care physicians in the service area, integration brings them together to achieve common goals. Today, reimbursement scenarios are causing many OB/GYNs to seek to serve as primary care providers. Physicians in their solo practices rarely get together to discuss common goals and strategies. They are too busy taking care of their patients and running their practices. By coming together in an integration effort, physicians and their hospitals can begin working together to form a primary care base.

Integration can lead to strength in managed care contracting. Many consultants believe that the payors want one-stop shopping when contracting with providers. This makes sense in that the payors would need to spend less time selling, managing, and administering numerous contracts, but in reality they can save far more money by "dividing and conquering" physicians, relying on physicians' fear of being left out if they do not sign a contract. Integrating can give leverage back to physicians. Integration through joint equity is a new technique and therefore is innovative. It also addresses all the reasons acquisitions tend to fail, and therefore can also be considered for this reason.

Integration in the joint equity model can also align incentives. Because everyone has a vested interest in making the integration effort succeed, everyone should be working to make decisions that are in the best interest of the health system. Aligning incentives includes putting physicians at risk for generating revenues, managing expenses, and caring about the bottom line so that their equity in the organization continues to grow.

Integration also improves access for the community because the hospital and physicians have incentives to grow the business, which includes serving all communities in the service area, expanding the service area, reducing outmigration and keeping patients in the service area, and adding new services.

The Risk of Doing Nothing

It makes good business sense to pursue an integration strategy. There are risks of doing nothing (that is, maintaining the status quo): loss of competitive advantage, loss of ability to lower health care delivery system costs, ability for payors to split the provider community, and inability to create integrated health care delivery system. The greatest risk is that someone else will integrate for you. There has been a proliferation of OB/GYN specialty care networks over the past few years and, although a few have demonstrated tenacity in a tumultuous market, niche players continue to make inroads. Many markets are just now coming to realize that the old system is not going to last. Tertiary systems are expanding their boundaries, especially for primary care services, as they attempt to increase their market share and so replace their declining admissions. Integration at the local level can prevent a tertiary provider (which usually has deeper pockets than a community hospital) from this type of expansion.

Lack of integration keeps providers in their separate organizations working for their own survival. It prevents them from being able to get together and work to drive costs out of the system and thus be competitive from a pricing perspective.

In addition, providers are not able to negotiate with payors as a group, thus allowing the payors to split the provider community. The payors will go to each provider with a contract favorable to the payor and play the providers one against the other. In the past, most providers have been worried about getting locked out of contracts and thus have been willing to sign unfavorable contracts to ensure access to patients. On top of this, most independent providers do not have the expertise to evaluate contracts beyond what the fee schedule of capitation rate is. An example of this is how coordination of benefits is handled. Another example is a capitation contract that requires a provider to bill separately for screening exams like mammography. This usually works to the advantage of the payors as the providers either forget or just don't know that these revenues are due them.

Lastly, providers will not have the ability to create an integrated health care delivery system. Many providers argue this point. In reality what is in existence now is an organized delivery system. Most communities have all the basic needs of primary care services, some degree of specialty care services, long-term care, pharmacy services, and the like. For more specialized services, referrals are made to larger communities that have tertiary and quaternary services including transplant, radiation therapy, bone marrow transplant, and others. However, these are not integrated; they are separate legal entities, have separate information systems, have separate financial and clinical systems, are under separate governance systems, and usually only "talk" to each other when referrals and sometimes utilization review are involved. Thus they are organized, but not integrated. Integration begins to occur when the legal, financial, clinical, and governance barriers are removed.

CRITICAL SUCCESS FACTORS OF PHYSICIAN INTEGRATION

Physicians are looking for three critical success factors: income, equity, and governance. Failure to address all three sets up an integration effort for failure.

The number one issue for physicians is income. Physicians have been through thirty plus years of training and provide an extremely specialized service. They feel, rightly so, that they should be adequately compensated for their services. The compensation strategy of any integration effort must be agreed to by physicians, and so must be fair to all concerned. This includes base salary, bonuses, and fringe benefits.

Most, although not all, physicians want to and are used to being the owner of the business. This does not disappear when they are looking to become part of an integration effort, whether it's a clinic without walls, a physician-hospital organization, or a joint equity group practice. Physicians like to know that at the end of the day, they have been able to build something of value, and that when they are ready to retire or move on, that they can sell their "sweat equity." Physicians involved in the sale of their practice during early integration efforts had their equity stripped away, albeit with cash as compensation. However, physician satisfaction in these situations was compromised.

Physicians are used to making decisions, year after year, day after day, patient after patient. Physicians want to be part of the decision-making process regardless of their income and regardless of their equity position. Physician satisfaction is likely to be low in circumstances where the physician has little or no voice or governance.

The traditional physician acquisition scenario and the new joint equity model are compared in Table 12.1. Keep the three critical success factors in mind when reviewing the comparisons.

CHECKLIST OF LEGAL ISSUES FOR JOINT VENTURES

Putting together a joint venture is not a simple process. It is more than simply filing articles of incorporation with the state and opening your doors for business. It takes careful planning and attention to the details as discussed thus far in this chapter. Following is a comprehensive, though not exclusive, list of issues that must be considered. It is wise to engage professional assistance to help navigate the federal, state, and local legal aspects of joint ventures.

Acquisition Model	Joint Equity Model
Mentality is to cash out	Vision is to be business partners
Learning to be efficient	Leveraging efficiencies
Employment relationship	Equity or ownership relationship
Salary compensation	Production-based compensation
Incentives are minimal or missing	Incentives based on productivity, performance, group financial goals, growth
Governance minimal or missing	Governance required

Table 12.1. Traditional Physician Acquisition Versus New Joint Equity Model.

- Medicare/Medicaid fraud and abuse
- Self-referral restrictions (federal and state)
- Antitrust
- Tax exemption
- Certificate of need
- Corporate practice of medicine
- Insurance regulations
- Physician practice parameters
- Medical malpractice liability
- Employee Retirement Income Security Act (ERISA)
- Reimbursement
- Securities issues
- Governance
- Other

WHICH MODEL IS RIGHT FOR YOU?

Choosing the right model is a critical first step. Often, an administrator will attend a seminar or read a book and think that a certain model is the exact solution for his or her situation and will work feverishly to make that model a reality. Later on, when the project fails, or is never completed due to resistance from the other parties, a self-examination will reveal that the form did not achieve the strategy. Whether this was due to local politics, or to lack of education, or to being ahead of your time is not really the point, although finding out the causes of failure can put the process back on track.

As discussed at the beginning of this chapter, form follows function and function follows strategy. Trying to implement a staff model when the physicians desire to remain autonomous is doomed to failure. Developing a PHO when the physicians desire to have a common voice in contract negotiations has a chance for success. Developing a PHO to keep out managed care and keep physician incomes high is unlikely to succeed. Creating a joint equity group practice to achieve clinical integration and streamline operations has a chance to succeed. The key is that the strategic objective will determine what functions need to be performed, which in turn drives which form may be most appropriate.

Formulating a Strategy

The first step is to determine what providers want to achieve. It is often helpful to have one or more educational seminars as part of these meetings, where providers can learn what is happening at the national, state, and local level and learn what are the driving forces behind these changes. Physicians will also want to know what other physicians have done, and whether they are successful. This may require several meetings in which the hospital and physicians openly discuss what they want.

During these discussions, keep track of the physicians' and hospital's goals. Put them on a flip chart and post them on the walls for everyone to see. This open discussion will help determine common themes, who will be interested in what level of integration, who will be a champion, and who will be counterproductive. Out of these goals and objectives, a strategy can be formulated.

Determining Function

After going through the process of determining why you are pursuing a physician integration strategy, the next step is to determine which functions need to be provided to meet these strategic objectives.

Most often, an integrated delivery system focuses on a primary care physician services network strategy. But this is not always the case. Sometimes the focus is to provide occupational medicine services, or to enhance contract negotiations and management. Sometimes the focus is on providing physician practice management services. Each market will be different, with different needs, different political circumstances, different geography, and so on.

Selecting a Form

The form can be one of the entry models (including management service bureaus [MSBs] and clinics without walls [CWWs]), transition models (including physician-hospital organizations [PHOs] and independent physician associations [IPAs]), or group practice models (including staff equity models, independent physician group practices, joint equity group practices, and asset MSOs), or a variation thereof. A PHO is a good choice for an entity whose function is to be a contracting vehicle, but not for providing management services. An MSO is a good choice for providing management services, but not for achieving clinical integration. A joint equity model is a good choice for achieving clinical integration, but not for maintaining physician autonomy. And so on.

The form can take many legal variations. The most commonly selected legal structure is that of the limited liability company (LLC). It is selected because it functions like a partnership for tax purposes and avoids the double taxation of a corporation, and at the same time functions like a corporation in terms of limiting the liability of the shareholders to their investment. In addition, the LLC is a flexible organizational structure that can be modified over time to meet the changing demands of the environment.

Different functions may lead to different forms. For example, if the functions being provided are occupational medicine services rather than primary care services, then it is likely that Medicare and Medicaid are more than minor payors. A form could be selected that otherwise might be restricted under the proposed Stark II law.

HOSPITAL-PHYSICIAN SYMBIOSIS

Hospitals have always depended on local physicians for patients. This is not going to change anytime soon. The only way a patient can be admitted or have tests ordered is through the written orders of physicians with the appropriate licenses and credentials. Thus, a hospital has a vested interest in ensuring that the community it serves has an appropriate number of physicians in each specialty to meet the demand for services. At the same time, hospitals are very expensive to build and operate. Because physicians do not have the financial capability of a hospital, they depend on the availability of the local resources (that is, ancillary services such as imaging, lab, and pharmacy) of the hospital for a significant portion of their revenue.

Physician Demand

How does a hospital know what is the right mix of physicians? Sophisticated software applications and extensive databases can be used to predict what the service needs will be for a given population. These applications use historical information as a baseline and assumptions about the future to predict future utilization. These predictions take into account factors such as age and gender mix, geographic location, managed care penetration, and more. Thus, the assumptions as well as the formulae they impact are critical.

As part of this process, hospitals must do the following:

- Define the service area. This is typically done using historical data such as inpatient admissions.
- Determine what will happen in the future.
- Plug the assumptions into the software program.
- Review the results for reasonableness.
- Interpret the results.

Most hospitals profile their service areas to determine the need for physician services by specialty. In this era of managed care, primary care physicians are most often in demand.

Primary Care Physicians

Primary care is usually defined as general practice, family practice, general internal medicine, and pediatrics. There is some debate as to whether to include obstetrics and gynecology as primary care or specialty care because it really is a crossover between the two. Regardless, it can be argued that having sufficient primary care physicians is a key to survival for hospitals. In addition, it may become more important in the future to concentrate on services for women, such as OB/GYN, because of the mother's role in decisions regarding the family's health care.

SUMMARY

Catering to women may be key to a hospital's financial future because it is women who choose which health plan (and thereby which providers) the family will use. Meeting women's needs includes having sufficient female OB/GYN physicians in the right locations so that women will access them. In order for a hospital to position itself to receive the referrals from these OB/GYN and related primary care physicians, many hospitals are seeking ways to partner, or integrate, with physicians. The joint equity model, described in some detail in this chapter, is one option that is demonstrating success in many local markets.

Notes

1. "Carve-Out Network Allows OB/GYNs to Maintain a Place in Prepaid Dollar Stream." *Managed OB/GYN: The Capitation Series.* Marietta, Ga.: National Health Information Service, 1997, p. 4.

2. Scarbeck, K. "OB/GYNs Turn to Management Firms." *OB/GYN News,* June 1, 1997, pp. 1, 48.

3. Medici Healthcare Consulting of Princeton, LLC. "Profile of OB/GYN Practice." *Economic Impact.* Washington, D.C.: Department of Medical Practice Economics, American College of Obstetricians and Gynecologists, 1998, pp. 107–109.

CHAPTER THIRTEEN

Practicing Care
The Nurse Practitioner Model

Cathy Hoot

Cathy Hoot is a writer and consultant in marketing and
sales as well as physician recruitment and retention in
Nashville. She has served on the advisory board of the
American College of Medical Staff Development. She was
previously director of medical staff development for
HealthTrust, which merged with Columbia/HCA.

The American Academy of Nurse Practitioners defines
a nurse practitioner as a "registered nurse with advanced education
and clinical competency necessary for the delivery of primary health
and medical care." Advanced education, such as a master's degree,
gives nurse practitioners the clinical expertise to provide health care
for individuals of all ages. Many of the available nurse practitioner
training programs offer specialty training in areas such as obstetrics,
pediatrics, and mental health. The settings they practice in range from
freestanding primary care clinics, to school or occupational health
clinics, to hospital outpatient clinics and emergency rooms.

This chapter examines why the nurse practitioner practice model's
has risen in popularity over the past few years. We see that nurses have
been educated to be more relationship- and care-oriented, more likely

to spend time with patients, to listen, and to treat the patient as a person—not a number, a disease, or an ailment. They have the reputation for bringing a holistic, patient-focused perspective to any health care setting. The average consumer, and particularly the female consumer, has begun to migrate toward this model because of a perceived higher concentration of sensitivity and responsiveness. Most patients, male and female, would like to have a personal guide through the health care maze and sometimes circuitous route back to health.

STRENGTHS OF THE NURSE PRACTITIONER MODEL

Colleen Conway-Welch, professor and dean of the Vanderbilt University School of Nursing, likens the role of the nurse practitioner to that of a trapeze artist: "Patients are moving from sites of care to other sites of care in order to meet the full spectrum of their health care needs. It is in the transition from one site to the next where patients may fall if no one is properly managing each link along the continuum of care. Nurse practitioners are also very effective safety nets because they can provide a patient-sensitive guide to help the patient make the next connection."

This metaphor demonstrates that the nurse practitioner model can create an opportunity to meet patients' individual needs, keep them from falling through the cracks, and capitalize on the nurse practitioner's strengths as a care giver. Do patients like to be guided through the health care process? Consumer information indicates that they do when it means proper management of their health care needs and services, continuity in the care they receive, getting follow-up from their care giver, and enjoying a high level of communication between patient and provider. There is ample evidence that today's patients not only expect this kind of health care, but seek out the clinics and providers, physician or otherwise, who can provide it.

One good example of this is the Columbia Advanced Practice Nurse Associates (CAPNA), a clinic of four nurse practitioners on Manhattan's Upper East Side. The clinic was established by Mary Mundinger, dean of Columbia University's School of Nursing in New York. The number of patients selecting CAPNA for their health care has grown steadily, mostly due to word of mouth advertising about the staff's personal touch and the healing environment of the clinic. CAPNA has proven that patients, especially women, will choose a nurse practitioner for their primary care. It has also demonstrated that payors will reimburse for that care at a rate that can keep the organization viable. After the Oxford Health Plans agreed in 1996 to pay CAPNA nurses the same as physicians for primary care services, other HMOs followed their lead.[1]

The strengths of the nurse practitioner practice model are evident:

- *Relationship-centered health care.* Its providers are relationship-centered by both natural orientation and training.

- *Woman to woman.* A high percentage of nurse practitioners are female, and many women today prefer a female health care provider.

- *Provide what most female patients seek.* The model brings sensitivity into the equation of what women are looking for: access and convenience, collaborative and sensitive health care, personalized education and information. Women want to make informed choices regarding their health and the health of their family. The nurse practitioner, as an experienced health care professional and empathetic educator, can help women to make informed decisions with confidence.

- *Fits the "niche" strategy.* The niche strategy is a business development area that is increasing as reimbursement patterns vary and customers demand services targeted to problems that are age- or sex-related.

- *Higher patient satisfaction.* Patient satisfaction usually is higher when more time is spent with the patient. Nurse practitioners typically can spend more time with each patient because they see fewer patients per day than most primary care physicians.

- *Has application in underserved markets.* In rural markets physician recruitment is difficult and primary care providers are not always available to provide easily accessible, local health care. A number of studies have shown that nurse practitioners can handle from 85 to 95 percent of all primary care health issues. These studies also show that the quality of care is similar to that provided by physicians in primary care practices.[2]

- *Strong focus on patient education and empowerment.* There is a strong focus on providing education for the patient and the patient's family. This can have the effect of not only improving overall health status, but in helping them make appropriate choices about self-care and about using health care services and resources.

PROBLEMS OF THE NURSE PRACTITIONER MODEL

Still, the practical application of this model in today's health care business environment is less than perfect. There are problems in this model, some of which stem from its strengths. For example, like a large number of physicians, many nurse practitioners lack understanding of the financial and operations aspects of health care. Fortunately for nurse practitioners, their understanding of the business side of health care is not a burning issue for the patients. Patients appreciate care and concern, not a focus on cost-consciousness.

The weaknesses of the nurse practitioner model include the following:

- *Difficulty in keeping the practice financially viable.* A nurse practitioner would have difficulty keeping a practice viable if he or she doesn't have a practice schedule similar to most primary care physicians. A primary care physician such as a family practitioner will average about 93 to 130 patients per week.[3] Nurse practitioner practice patterns indicate a lower patient volume than most doctors and it is realistic to say that they average much less than ninety-three patient visits per week. Because a nurse practitioner could not have a financially viable practice with only eighteen patients per day, the stand-alone nurse practitioner model, like the physician practice model, would probably have to be an assembly-line situation.

- *Limitations imposed by licensing and payor restrictions.* Practitioners have to be very aware and concerned about billing within an appropriate range and scope of services, not only from a health plan and reimbursement standpoint but also within the full diagnostic and treatment capabilities allowed by the state in which they are licensed.

- *Provider's limited exposure to the business side of health care.* Nurse practitioners may be desirable providers as far as patients are concerned, but they may lack knowledge as well as an understanding of and a true buy-in to the business model that keeps a health care company viable. This could cause a financial glitch that may have an impact on the organization's financial viability and ultimately the practitioner's livelihood.

The nurse practitioner has been trained for many roles relating to the patient: interviewer, educator, skilled health care provider, case manager, and consultant. Being a business person is one role that most nurse practitioners are not trained for and usually have only a minimal interest in and exposure to. Their business has always been comprehensive care of the patient but their focus must broaden to include an understanding of how to keep a practice financially viable.

BOLSTERING THE BUSINESS SIDE

Roxanne Spitzer, chief operating officer of the Vanderbilt Medical Group Network, acknowledges that nurse practitioners often lag behind doctors in having an extensive knowledge of the business aspect of the delivery of health care. And because most doctors, though clinically well trained, are woefully underexposed to the specifics of creating and operating a successful business, this indicates an even greater threat and disadvantage to the average nurse practitioner's practice. In today's environment of shrinking reimbursement patterns and cost-reducing measures, the nurse practitioner needs a business perspective and understanding commensurate with the tight budget constraints of today's health care delivery systems.

Medical training institutions must capture the secrets of producing physicians, nurse practitioners, and all other health care providers who can competently treat patients while delighting them with their concern and communication—all within the framework of a financial reality that is lean and mean. Being lean and mean requires financial viability that spans both the revenue and expense side of the medical practice. Managed care can complicate this issue by making revenues harder to come by and expenses more difficult to manage because it is not only managed care, but managed costs. Health care must be high quality, multifaceted, comprehensive, and cost-effective in every managed care organization (MCO). MCOs have a strong incentive to find the most efficient combination of health care professionals to provide care to their patient population. This mix often includes nonphysician providers such as nurse practitioners or nurse midwives.

In any health care environment, the clinician and the operations manager have two very different purposes. The clinician provides the services and the operations manager is ultimately responsible for collecting payment for those services. Both must collaborate to keep the organization in business. Jaynelle F. Stichler of the Stichler Group describes this necessary partnership: "The goals of almost all health care organizations are generally to ensure quality patient outcomes and a positive financial environment so the organization remains a viable entity. The discrepancy in power between the clinical nurse and the manager is balanced when each recognizes and values the importance of the other's role in fulfilling the organization's overall mission."[4]

THE NURSE PRACTITIONER MODEL PAYS OFF

In an ever-tightening managed care environment, collaboration is extremely important and creates a health care entity that can function well and thrive financially. When it exists, there are opportunities in today's marketplace for the nurse practitioner practice model.

Roxanne Spitzer indicated that the best practice opportunity for a nurse practitioner is one that allows the nurse practitioner to practice interdependently and intradependently with other providers, the payor (or health plan), and the patient. Spitzer considers a capitated system to be the best example of this. The emphasis is on a collaborative effort among all health care providers, both primary care and specialists. Additional emphases are preventive medicine and educating patients on ways to restore health and to stay well. The capitation model is where demand management and disease management really translate to the bottom line. The investment of the nurse practitioner's time and expertise has a return for the system and the patient. Finally, there is a true alignment of incentives.

For example, under capitation, accessibility and quick response to a patient's call or request can be rewarded with a healthier patient who will use the capitated plan's resources and providers more prudently. In contrast, under a fee-for-service setting the time and steps necessary to accomplish this kind of response and communication—taking a patient's call, retrieving the chart, and discussing a specific problem and possible solution with the patient—may even be considered downtime because it may reduce the number of patients seen and is not specifically a billable activity.

Spitzer suggested a second model that is also an example of a practice situation that allows the nurse practitioner to practice interdependently and intradependently with the health plan and the patient. The nurse practitioner is employed to be an in-house primary care provider for a company's employees and usually sees the employees in or close to the work site. This could be financially advantageous for both the company and the nurse practitioner. The practitioner doesn't have the pressure of the business side or productivity issues of the practice, and the employer may see a reduction in overall health care benefits costs and perhaps even higher employee productivity and a reduction in employee absenteeism. If this model were staffed to accommodate employees' family members, there may be added advantages for both the company and the employed nurse practitioner.

ISSUES AND OPPORTUNITIES

There is a strong case for the nurse practitioner practice model and the settings that may offer the most opportunity for the provider and the payor, but there are issues and obstacles when it comes to creating successful practices:

- The nurse practitioner may resist changing behaviors and attitudes as necessary to assure the success of the practice.
- The nurse practitioner may feel that to be concerned with making money, or breaking even, is somehow divergent to a commitment to focus on patient care.
- Few markets are capitated. How can the nurse practitioner's practice potential translate in the interim economic strategies before capitation is a reality? What if it is never a reality in the market?
- Inappropriate billing, or poor understanding of billing parameters, is very dangerous for the long-term financial viability of any provider—and ignorance, laziness, or having a patient-oriented focus instead of a bottom-line focus are not acceptable excuses for these missteps.
- By focusing on the bottom line, are we in danger of losing or compromising client intimacy?

Despite these issues, nurse practitioners are becoming more widely accepted and requested than ever before. They all want to work in a setting that allows them to exercise their highest values of service and competency and also compensates them well for the job they do. Most want to help patients get better and maybe even delight them with the care they receive. Colleen Conway-Welch says that patients are delighted by the following:

- Being listened to by a well-educated, competent health care professional

- Having an appropriate amount of time spent with them

- Being considered and treated as a person with a name and a health care challenge, not as number, disease, or ailment

- Having little things remembered about them from one visit to the next

- Being given educational materials that address the mind-body continuum, not just their disease or ailment

- Being given the appropriate diagnosis and treatment

- Receiving quality treatment with minimal out-of-pocket cost

Conway-Welch and Spitzer also mentioned specific techniques that could delight patients:

- Carry a portable phone at all times to increase accessibility and response to patients.

- Provide a key pad to input questions the patient may ask during a visit. Be prepared to bring them up with the patient for discussion or follow-up either via phone or during the next visit.

- Have a list of helpful Internet Web site addresses relating to something the patient mentioned as a concern or interest.

- Add a module to the practice management system to allow input of comments or personal information that staff or clinicians can mention when the patient calls or comes in. For example, How was your daughter's birthday party last week? What special plans do you have for your anniversary this month? Is your little boy over the cold you mentioned last time you were in? Are you enjoying your new job? Congratulations on your promotion at work!

- Send congratulatory cards to patient and family members as appropriate.

There are virtually hundreds of little ways the practice can delight patients. All relate to listening well, responding quickly, exceeding expectations, and reaffirming their sense of "person" and importance in a business environment that is becoming more and more depersonalized and disappointing to many.

For some practitioners and doctors in private practice who may have essentially a break-even practice now, implementing a variety of these patient delights could make a huge contribution to long-term viability of the practice. In addition, Spitzer suggests another business development strategy: specialty niches that relate to the large numbers of aging female and male baby boomers. Problems such as incontinence or impotence are specialty areas that could provide the practitioner with patients who are willing to pay for services tailored to these special needs. Generational issues facing older women, such as aging parents or dealing with difficult adolescents, also create business opportunities in the mental health arenas. Spitzer cautions that although these specialty areas could increase the financial viability of a practice, the patient must still be considered a person rather than a niche.

In addition, there are opportunities for nurse practitioners in a variety of markets:

- Freestanding primary care clinics
- Home health settings
- Occupational health clinics
- Inpatient and long-term care facilities
- Emergency rooms
- School-based clinics
- Employer-based clinics

SUMMARY

Nurse practitioners are often requested and favored by many health care consumers today and they can be an important part of any health care delivery system. Physicians, practice administrators, health care leaders, and executives of hospitals and other health care facilities should consider including nurse practitioners as primary care providers and as specialty care providers.

By being innovative in their attention to the patient and to the business side of health care, the nurse practitioners of the present and future can be assured of their place in any existing or future health care delivery system. After all, the things that keep patients satisfied and payors placated are things that nurses and nurse practitioners have always been better at than just about any other health care provider group.

Notes

1. Gregory, S. S., and Campbell, J. "No Docs Allowed." *People,* Sept. 21, 1998, pp. 117–118.
2. Sackett, D. L., and others. "The Burlington Randomized Trial of Nurse Practitioners: Health Outcomes of Patients." *Annals of Internal Medicine,* 1997, *17,* S165; Spitzer, W. O., and others. "The Nurse Practitioner Revisited." *New England Journal of Medicine,* 1996, *310*(16), 50–51.
3. Practice Support Resources. *Practice Management STATS Quick Reference Guide: Update 1998.* Practice Support Resources, 1998.
4. Association of Women's Health, Obstetric and Neonatal Nurses. "Developing Collaborative Relationships: Balancing Professional Power in the Health Care Environment." *Lifelines,* June 1998, pp. 19–21.

CHAPTER FOURTEEN

Employer Strategies: Women in the Workforce

Genie James
Holly E. Owens

> *Holly E. Owens is proposal request team manager for*
> *TCS Management Group, Inc., in Brentwood, Tennessee.*
> *Her professional experience includes marketing and*
> *writing for health management companies.*

———

W hy should health care providers examine women's health as a component of their employer strategies? Very simply, providers are competing to differentiate themselves in the marketplace and to protect themselves from market share erosion. Because, as already established, women control most of the health care decisions, they are a force that has an impact on market share. When a provider system is developing an employer-directed strategy, the importance of the female consumer is magnified because now she is an employee.

Increasing evidence substantiates the importance of addressing women's health as integral to the aggressive employer-directed strategy. In July 1998, the Department of Health and Human Services (HHS) released the first comprehensive report on the health and well-being of America's working women. It profiled key statistics for the more than sixty million women who are part of the American labor force, using data from the Departments of Health and Human Services, Labor, and Commerce.[1] The statistics provide an important baseline for learning more about the needs of working women and opportunities to improve their health.

Since 1950 the labor force has increased at least 170 percent, so that today more than one-half of adult women work. During that period, women as a proportion of the labor force doubled from one-fourth to nearly one-half of workers. The report describes the sociodemographics, household characteristics, and health of women according to workforce status and job conditions, with comparative data for men.[2] Today, more women are working and they are continuing to work through and beyond their childbearing years. By the millennium, fifty million U.S. women will be at least fifty years old. Meeting the long-ignored health concerns of these women will be a transforming experience for those charged with designing health benefits plans and models for the delivery of care.

OPPORTUNITIES AHEAD

How can a provider system work with the employer to do the following?

- Assess the health risks associated with employees
- Anticipate the financial exposure related to treating women's health concerns, including osteoporosis, cardiovascular disease, depression and cancer
- Target the female employee as pivotal to a proactive strategy for health management that has the potential of reducing medical claims costs

The answer begins with harnessing the data and then translating it into meaningful health management information. Provider systems have a real opportunity to triage decision support data to position themselves as a key partner to the employer who is asking for the tools to reduce medical claims costs. The question now becomes, How do hospitals and employers work together to target the female employee in order to receive the greatest return on investment of resources?

As health care costs continue to rise, and there is every indication they will, employers will become increasingly concerned with ways to curtail them. According to Robert S. Galvin, "The most recent KPMG Peat Marwick Report shows premium increases of 3.3 percent through March, 1998. . . . It will take a combination of cost increases consistently greater than 5 to 7 percent, accompanied by a softening in top line revenue growth, for the mass of employers to get concerned enough about profitability to take on some of the tough issues in health care."[3]

Recent news headlines cite HMO horror stories as backlash builds against the managed care sector, which has gotten the reputation for collecting premiums but limiting access to care, most notably for specialist services. Furthermore, educated consumers with access to the Internet are taking more active roles in managing their health care. For many, the perceived promise of managed care—to simultaneously enhance efficiency and quality of care—has fallen short of expectations. The resulting public distress has attracted the attention of state and national legislatures intent on reforming the sector and is likely to heat up further as the next election approaches.

Compounding an increasingly negative public and consumer perception, corporate America is becoming more aggressive on the same issues as health insurance premiums continue to rise in the recovery phase of the pricing cycle. After achieving measurable cost savings from the late 1980s to the mid-1990s that were passed on to employers via dramatic reductions in insurance premium inflation, managed care organizations (MCOs) combating margin declines have been forced to raise premiums well ahead of general economic inflation levels over the past few years.[4]

Employers are now seeing that managed care has not effectively reduced their health care costs. Herein lies an opportunity for the health system looking for ways to meet the needs of local employers and subsequently protect market share. This opportunity is disease management or, with a more positive spin, health management.

In fact, one of the toughest issues in health care today is the need to shift from sick care to well care. For the provider community, it has been difficult to justify a commitment to preventive medicine because there is very little financial return from it. However, employers are demonstrating that they want a healthier workforce and they are not waiting for providers to show them how to get one.

Several factors are motivating the large, self-insured employer to demand that primary prevention become an integral component of primary care services:

- Continuing concern about ongoing increases in health care costs and the need for effective interventions before disease or acute episodes occur

- A growing awareness of the potential cost savings associated with accident prevention, injury control, and stress reduction

- Increased employee interest in information about improving personal health behaviors[5]

Suddenly the hospital can have an enthusiastic new customer base that is ready and able to contract for health promotion services. The employer's motivation to buy is not soft: it is the potential for significant financial savings that drives them to encourage healthy lifestyles for their workers.[6]

A great example is the Stanford Corporate Health Program of the Stanford University School of Medicine.[7] Since 1984, the goal of this program has been to develop and evaluate innovative medical and health promotion programs in the workplace as an integral part of managed care for both purchasers and providers. Under the direction of Kenneth R. Pelletier, the research program involves a unique collaboration between the Stanford Center and twenty-one corporations, including Aetna, AT&T, Bank of America, IBM, Motorola, and Pacific Bell. Among the research and development areas in progress in the Stanford program are the following:

- Behavioral management of hypertension and coronary heart disease

- Computer or telephone health delivery systems

- Early cancer screening, especially mammography for women

- Smoking cessation

- Health promotion programs to reach minorities, dependents, and retirees

- Alcohol and substance abuse programs

- Dietary and nutritional counseling

- Physical fitness and back-saver programs

- AIDS prevention and policy information
- Applications of meditation and relaxation for stress management
- Reaching small or remote worksites
- Comprehensive program evaluation

Other companies are working to shift the burden to the employee by making wellness fun. Cosmetics maker Avon Products, Inc., in New York has revived a program encouraging its sales representatives to compete in regional, national, and global five-kilometer walks and ten-kilometer runs. About eighty John Hancock Financial Services employees ran the 1999 Boston Marathon, sponsored by the company. About 177,498 runners from 5,861 companies ran in the 1998 Chase Corporate Challenge, a sixteen-city, three-and-a-half-mile event sponsored by Chase Manhattan Bank. A fourth of Nike's five thousand employees traverse trails on the corporate campus in Beaverton, Oregon.[8]

As the employer community begins to demand a more aggressive and long-term strategy for reducing overall medical claims cost, the arena of preventive medicine and health management services takes on a new dimension of opportunity. It is still important to remember that health management is a new business for most hospitals and health systems and—although many have branched into this area via their occupational medicine programs, worksite wellness services, and community health initiatives—few have been able to position these services as much more than goodwill cost centers.

ALLIANCES FOR HEALTH STATUS MANAGEMENT

Some hospitals and health systems have begun to address the demand for health management services via loose community alliances. Others have taken a disease management approach to moving toward health management opportunities. Frequently they get no further than agreeing on philosophy, but a few have proven that collaboration can actually deliver.

Cindy Nayer, president of the River City Partnership, promotes creating what she calls "the invisible fabric of support" across a community. In 1998, Eli Lilly Company contacted the Missouri Governor's Council on Physical Fitness and Health to seek counsel on creating a women's coalition to advance health care decision making. Nayer, as chair of the council, had raised awareness of women's health issues. She was asked to build and chair a coalition of organizations that could focus on leadership and advocacy, beyond a one-time event. Because of her experience with such initiatives, Nayer was able to call on professional bonds created earlier. Invited to the coalition were hospital systems, managed care companies, pharmaceutical companies beyond Lilly, businesses, church groups, community action groups, and personal friends—competitive organizations who were encouraged to put aside their differences and create a launching event for a statewide advocacy group. The event was held in October 1998 and attracted over eight hundred women and twenty sponsoring organizations. Further, the coalition is serving as a catalyst for statewide initiatives in education, leadership, and advocacy.

Nayer's work deserves to be celebrated. However, although collaboration sounds good, too often no one individual or organization takes ownership of the process and drives the initiative from inception to the achievement of objectives. Collaborative ventures too often drain precious time and money.

THE DISEASE MANAGEMENT MODEL

Developing and implementing disease or health management initiatives is complicated. The goal of any program is to gain the ability to define and track the risk of disease across a population (membership) and to then develop systems of intervention through a comprehensive database systems approach. Critical steps in the process include the following:[9]

- *Selection of a high-yield disease state for program development.* High-yield disease programs are those that have measurable impact (both clinical and financial) and touch the lives of many persons, improving health status. These illnesses involve either chronic conditions that affect many members, or others (chronic or acute) that are less common but expensive to treat— the key being that appropriate therapeutic intervention offers the potential to have an impact on the disease.

- *Patient identification via use of stratification algorithms.* Gaining access to accurate claims and other medical data is critical, and having software systems capable of sifting through the data is equally important in identifying patients at risk of disease.

- *Formulation of treatment protocols via algorithms used by clinical experts.* Systems specialists, in conjunction with physician and allied clinical expert panels, develop sophisticated algorithms as assessment tools to create evidence-based guidelines. Disease profiles can be drilled down to the individual patient level, accounting for episodes of illness, severity of disease, comorbidities, and overall physical condition of the patient. This is essentially a risk screening process that includes automated analyses of patient health appraisals, medical claims history, quality of life issues, and compliance potential and issues.

- *Treatment intervention via buy-in of primary care providers.* Although all the components of any disease management model are important, the intervention step is arguably the most critical. In this function, the disease manager must coordinate all of the constituencies in an effort to achieve the desired outcome. There may be several players to coordinate: the key constituents are the patient and physician.

- *Coordinate care and monitor patients.* Nurse practitioner coordinators, pharmacists, dieticians, and other health professionals form a multidisciplinary team. They establish a rapport with the member or patient to achieve a buy-in such that long-term sustained behavior modification is accomplished, producing compliance with physician ordered treatment protocols. To be effective, the program must focus on management of the patient, not the disease, as chronic illness requires handling medical, psychosocial, and lifestyle issues.

- *Measure performance.* Disease managers use information systems to collect and analyze performance of the disease management program.

- *Use outcome studies to determine success of disease management programs.* This step provides a feedback loop, enabling continual refinement and improvement in the program. A successful program offers the potential for changing the course of disease, enhancing health status and outcomes. This improves quality of life and reduces overall medical delivery costs.

Can disease management services be leveraged to strengthen relationships with area employers? Absolutely! The Benfield Group, a national consulting firm based in St. Louis, has made a business of helping hospitals do just that. It works with hospitals and health systems to position prevention and wellness as an essential part of a health care organization's business model. It warns that too often employer-directed efforts fail because the hospital's approach is fragmented, reactionary, or not tied to meaningful, measured outcomes. Consequently, many hospitals do not reap the success they want because they are offering piecemeal services like screenings, classes, and health fairs without really targeting what they offer to the needs of their customers.

Because health management services have often been viewed as cost centers, many hospitals have chosen to outsource these functions. Diffusing the cost of start-up and sharing the risk for success is, for many provider systems, proving to be a much more fiscally responsible option for getting into the health management business. The Internet is also creating some new and cost-effective solutions for operationally delivering these health management services. Outsourcing to a responsible vendor has some operational merit as well. Several vendors today, including Staywell, Access Health, American Corporate Health, Carewise, Johnson & Johnson Health Care Systems, and Gordian Health Solutions, Inc., are attempting to establish a niche in the field of health management.

In choosing to outsource, it is important to identify a vendor whose services match your needs. If, for instance, you want to heighten visibility and awareness in your marketplace, you may choose to contract for educational materials. Topics available from Staywell, for instance, include the following:

- Computer fitness materials to keep people on the job
- Office ergonomics brochures to help employees avoid repetitive motion injuries
- A guide to forklift safety
- A guide to developing a low-stress work style
- Questions and answers about alcohol or drug use
- A personal action booklet and training kit on weight management

If, however, you want a spectrum of programs ranging from low cost and low impact to more costly with more impact, then you need to move beyond educational materials. One vendor positioning itself to be the hospital's choice for outsourcing these functions and becoming accountable for strategic business objectives is Gordian Health Solutions, Inc., the subject of the following section.

CASE STUDY: GORDIAN HEALTH SOLUTIONS, INC.

Gordian Health Solutions, Inc., has been providing results-oriented health management and Health Accountability Programs to employers since the mid-1980s with dramatic results. Gordian, based in Nashville, Tennessee, builds its success on a systematic approach to health management initiatives that is applicable in many circumstances. Gordian does the following:

1. Determines the historical factors contributing to claims costs through a comprehensive Retrospective Claims Analysis or Community Health Profile

2. Identifies high-risk and high-cost individuals through health risk assessments

3. Quantifies the participation of targeted high-risk individuals (through monitoring or physician referral)

4. Tracks compliance and participation in the health management program

5. Documents the reduction in medical claims costs

Gordian has developed a Strategic Employer Initiative that is grounded in the belief that informed decisions and actions are better than uninformed. It's an obvious business principle, but the fact is that many hospitals and health systems implement health promotion or management programs based on a general, common sense knowledge of their population's risks—and then they hope for a little luck. The problem with this is that even if program results seem successful, there is no substantive way to measure or gauge it. Too much time and money is wasted on initiatives that are either ill-founded or insufficient. Instead, Gordian's simple recommendation is this: gather as much information about a target population as possible, identify the problem areas, and then start thinking about ways to alleviate the identified risks.

Health management information is the beginning of the solution. Gordian provides this by looking at the historical claims costs of an employee population through its Retrospective Claims Analysis or by analyzing hospital billing data to determine the cost savings potential for a community population via its Community Health Profile. Unique to the Gordian approach is that it goes way beyond simply analyzing where the checks for health care costs were written. It projects the potential costs associated with various response strategies that the employer might take, from a minimal strategy of simply providing the employee with health management information to a very aggressive and intensive individualized high-risk disease management program.

Gordian's methodology is rooted in pragmatism and a measurable return on investment. In this way, Gordian can be a viable partner for those hospitals or health systems evaluating whether to "make, rent or buy." At the time of this writing, Gordian had just finalized a strategic partnership with the National Business Coalition on

Health, the umbrella agency for one hundred business coalitions serving multiple employers responsible for approximately thirty million covered lives. This relationship provides ample evidence of a target customer very willing to buy.

RETURN ON INVESTMENT

Although employer demand for health management information and services may be creating a greater incentive for provider involvement, the reality is that a commitment to this approach will not immediately show up on a balance sheet. Providers are motivated to move into this arena because of their need to protect market share, differentiate themselves in a competitive environment, and formalize relationships with local employers. Providers who consider a commitment to health management services must recognize that they can no longer exploit the inherent financial returns of a sick-care system. The consumer (the employer) and the end user (the female employee) are demanding value. Value has previously been defined in this text as "cost plus quality plus patient satisfaction equals value."

As we move into the new millennium, employers will be examining all the components contributing to health care costs. Providers will be scrambling to define quality and then differentiate themselves accordingly. The female end-user will not be satisfied with a health care delivery system that meets only her sick-care needs. She wants to be healthy and she wants to be empowered to promote the health and well-being of those she loves and cares for. Altogether, it is obvious that if the efforts of hospitals and health systems to improve value are to ever pay off in the form of increased market share, then a women's health focus will be integral to any employer-directed strategy.

RECOMMENDED STRATEGIES

Those seeking corporate support for a women's wellness program are, according to Catherine Hawkes, assistant vice president of health management at CIGNA Corp. in Philadelphia, most likely to get it by approaching it like any other proposal in the business world. The wellness proposal will be most convincing, she believes, if it is based on data from authoritative sources, demonstrates potential costs and value and is presented succinctly and illustrated with relevant graphics. Here are a few guidelines:[10]

• Speak to corporate managers in their own language. Avoid terminology that sounds too "touchy-feely" for managerial ears.

"Retention, recruitment, attracting employees—that's what they want to hear in your crisp presentation," advises Jodi Fuller, senior program manager at mortgage lender Fannie Mae in Washington, D.C.

- Solicit senior managers' views on wellness and health management. "Talk about their own personal health and how they make health-seeking decisions," Hawkes suggests.

- Develop partnerships. Make it clear that forging partnerships with local hospitals can be advantageous for all concerned and can diffuse the costs of program administration for the employer, says Diana Murray, senior manager of group insurance plans at the Sara Lee Corp. in Chicago.

- Collaborate with health plans. The hospital should take the lead on helping employers and health plans to coordinate information.

- Educate women about preventive lifestyle measures. Investigate the potential to lower the cost of retiree benefits by reducing health risks.

- Benchmark successful programs. Find out which of your competitors sponsor women's wellness programs and what kind. Then develop a better one yourself.

- Anticipate resistance and expect to negotiate. "The concerns of senior-level managers who deal with board issues, shareholder value and succession planning are different from those of mid-level managers who are on the hook for creating the products and selling them," says Hawkes. Therefore, she advises, be sensitive to their probable "hot buttons." Are they concerned that wellness programs will occupy work time? That productivity will slip? Or that too many competing priorities exist already?

These guidelines are among the many creative approaches that can be used to build support for a women's health management program.

SUMMARY

Providers are aware of the importance of employer-directed strategies—and increasingly aware of the need to address women's health as an integral component of those strategies. The employer is readily viewed as an essential ally in any effort to reduce outmigration. It is also important for providers to acknowledge that the end user retains some degree of provider choice. To be successful, hospitals and health systems that are working toward market share differentiation must recognize the importance of courting the female employee and incorporate her need for a focus on health managment into an overall strategy for targeting area employers.

Notes

1. U.S. Department of Health and Human Services. *Women: Work and Health.* Washington, D.C.: U.S. Government Printing Office, 1998.

2. U. S. Department of Health and Human Services. *HHS Issues First Comprehensive Survey of Working Women's Health.* Report. 1999. Available from Sandra Smith of the NCHS Press Office, (301) 436–7551; from Fred Blosser of NIOSH, (202) 260–8519 or (800) 356–4674); or on the Internet at <http://www.cdc.gov/nchswww>.

3. Galvin, R. S. "Part II: What Do Employers Mean by 'Value'?" *Integrated Healthcare Report,* Oct. 1998, pp. 8–10.

4. Ray, J. M., and Sydnor, J. B. "Disease Management: The Future of Managed Care." *Disease Management Industry,* Apr. 12, 1999, p. 4.

5. James, G. *Making Managed Care Work: Strategies for Local Market Dominance.* Burr Ridge, Ill.: Irwin, 1997, p. 162.

6. Godar, K. (ed.). "Currents." *Hospitals & Health Networks,* July 5, 1994, p. 22.

7. The Stanford Corporate Health Program description is adopted from Pelletier, K. R. "Healthy People, Healthy Business." *Healthier Communities Summit,* 1995.

8. Beatty, S. "Work Week." *Wall Street Journal,* May 4, 1999, p. 1.

9. Ray and Sydnor, "Disease Management," pp. 13–15.

10. Voelker, R. "Seven Steps to Corporate Support for Women's Wellness." *Business & Health,* Special Report, Oct. 1998, pp. 15–16.

CHAPTER FIFTEEN

Creating Healing Environments for Women

Jaynelle F. Stichler

> *Jaynelle F. Stichler, D.N.S., is a principal in charge of the Healthcare Division at the Stichler Group, Inc., in San Diego. Her work is recognized throughout the nation and internationally in Australia, Mexico, Korea, Thailand, and Malaysia.*

The hospital is second nature to health care providers, but unnatural, frightening, and stressful to patients and their families. The language providers use is different, foreign sounding, and often secretive. Care givers provide services, but they sometimes do not seem to care. Many patients are nameless and are referred to by disease: "the gall bladder in bed two."

Further, our surroundings have physical components that have the potential to influence health. As an example, buildings may have toxic qualities from the use of fabrics, carpet, or paint that give off fumes that can be problematic for some. The light may be too intense or too dim to see properly and may interfere with our ability to work. A window may be facing the west sun, creating uncomfortable temperatures.

Buildings and rooms can evoke strong emotional messages as well. Some seem warm, inviting, comfortable, and feel like home; whereas others may seem very formal, imposing, or even intimidating. Government buildings may contribute to a much different feeling than a church, and hospitals may arouse different feelings than a health spa. We are constantly reacting and responding to our environment mentally, emotionally, and physically.

The environment in the hospital can make a difference in how quickly a patient recovers. It has been shown that patients who have hospital rooms with a window overlooking a small stand of trees have shorter recovery time (shorter length of stay, fewer medications for pain, and fewer negative notations in the nursing notes) than those whose windows provide a view of a brick wall.[1] Unfortunately, much of this research has been ignored. Perhaps it is because we have not truly believed that there is a relationship between environment and healing. But there is, so hospitals by nature of their purpose must have therapeutic, curative, and restorative physical settings. The environment must support professional practice while meeting the patient's and family's need for emotional and physical care.

Health is not a static phenomenon. It is a dynamic process to ensure a constructive and productive personal and social life,[2] a balancing process to ensure integrity of the self,[3] and an adapting process to stresses imposed on us by the external environment and internally by ourselves as we give meaning to life's experiences. Health is a feeling and a sense of wholeness and harmony with our environment. Florence Nightingale believed that a person's health (or illness) is the result of environmental influences.[4] The environment can restore health or impair the healing process. According to one expert, for every dimension of health there is a corresponding aspect of our built environment.[5] Environments can be sources of physical and mental stress, or they can facilitate relaxation, introspection, self-expression, and productivity.

Healing environments allow us to mobilize inner resources in the mind, body, and spirit that will enhance our ability to respond and react to internal and external forces that cause stress and distress: "When you are in a healing environment, you know it; no analysis is required. You somehow feel welcome, balanced, and at one with yourself and the world. You are relaxed and stimulated, reassured and invited to expand. You feel at home."[6] We can know a healing place subjectively when we find and experience it, but until recently we have not identified objective variables that actually create a healing environment.

ENVISIONING A HEALING ENVIRONMENT

Researchers have identified various environmental elements that have an effect on our health. Venolia proposed that healing environments do the following:[7]

- Stimulate positive awareness of ourselves—our mind, body, soul, past, and potential
- Enhance our connections with nature, culture, and people
- Allow for privacy and private space
- Do not harm us with toxic materials, stressful lighting, noise, or unbalanced temperatures
- Provide meaningful, varying stimuli
- Encourage relaxation with the use of peaceful sounds, calming colors, pleasant views, comfortable furniture, and a sense of harmony in the environment
- Allow choice and active participation with the environment such as the ability to open a window, control the lighting, or have options as to where to sit
- Provide balance of constancy and flexibility with changing of the seasons, the need to accommodate overnight guests, or the ability to rearrange furniture depending on changing needs
- Provide a sense of beauty

Until the 1990s, few hospitals considered these or other attributes in the design of hospitals or other health care settings. Hospitals are frequently designed with the input of professionals working with the architect, and often there is a conflict between what is needed to support professional practice and what is optimal to enhance the experience for the patient and family. As Carlson indicated, "Most hospitals today are built much like doctors' workshops and are more reminiscent of assembly-line manufacturing than temples of healing."[8]

ATTRIBUTES OF HEALING ENVIRONMENTS

But there is renewed interest in healing environments. Researchers at the Center for Health Design and the Picker Institute in Boston identified seven dimensions that are important to patients and families in the health care environment.[9] The patients and families indicated that a health care facility should facilitate connectedness to the staff and should be conducive to well-being; confidential and private; caring for both the patient and the family; considerate of patients' impairments; and close to nature.

Similar to these findings, Stichler and Weiss studied the health care customers' perception of quality and reported that the respondents indicated that quality hospitals are characterized as clean; orderly; safe; quiet; attractive; up to date; provide privacy; and allow the nurse or physician to be near you.[10]

Planetree, a nonprofit organization that led in the development of patient-centered principals, programs, and facility design, promoted the concept of healing environments by empowering patients to participate fully in their own healing process, providing open access to information, and promoting a holistic approach to health care that recognized the patient as an individual with physical, emotional, spiritual, and mental needs.

HEALING ENVIRONMENTS IN ACTION

Healing environments do exist. Not coincidentally, they often are linked to women's health. For example, when you walk into Wellspring for Women in Boulder, Colorado, you know immediately that it is a healing place. It is warm, inviting, charming, and it feels like home. Tapestries, quilts, dried flowers, and calming pictures create an environment of rest, peace, and harmony. As another example, the Elizabeth Blackwell Center in Columbus, Ohio, was created in a renovated church. The church lobby was transformed into a resource library complete with books and magazines on women's health. The library opens onto an enclosed patio, providing a sense of the outdoors coming inside the space. A pleasant retail space also serves as a welcoming area for visitors and provides a place to purchase note cards, books, and personal items of interest to women. The church sanctuary became a lecture room for classes and guest speakers providing the most current information about women's health issues. Offices for the clinical psychologists, nurse practitioners, physicians, and other health care providers were developed from the church school rooms and provide a place for individual counseling or support groups. Even a place for aerobics and other fitness and exercise programs was developed from the church gymnasium. It is truly a healing place, not only for the body but for the mind and spirit.

These healing environments did not occur by accident; they were planned. And the planning took into account the fact that most of the care for women is provided in the home setting by the woman herself and with the input of family and friends. Women's health services should reflect that level of comfort. They are predominantly provided in outpatient settings, women's health centers, women's clinics, family planning clinics, birthing centers, private physician's offices, multi-specialty medical groups, and a myriad of other places. Women's health is also provided in inpatient settings in maternity centers, GYN units, and other departments in acute care facilities.

A number of design elements and physical attributes can create spaces that enhance the healing process. Light, color, furnishings, smells, sound, and privacy are all important and can contribute to health.

Light

Light is symbolic in many faiths, and usually represents goodness, warmth, vision, creativity, and clarity. Conversely, darkness is symbolic of evil, fear, death, the unknown, coldness, and lack of vision. These ideas may not consciously enter in, but light—whether symbolic or actual—does play a role in health.

The absence of light in certain seasons and parts of the world can cause seasonal affective disorder (SAD), manifest as symptoms of fatigue, chronic irritability, frequent minor illnesses similar to cold or flu, and generalized muscle weakness. Light in an interior space also has an affect on mood, productivity, and health.

The harmful effects of sunlight and overexposure to ultraviolet (UV) light—skin cancer, sunburn, cataracts, and dry skin—are emphasized in the media. Yet it's important to bear in mind that UV light has many benefits also. UV light can increase protein metabolism, lessen fatigue, stimulate white blood cell production, increase the release of endorphins, lower blood pressure, elevate mood, and generally promote healing. Light can be therapeutic, as in its use to decrease bilirubin levels in newborns or in the use of ultraviolet light to treat psoriasis.

Unfortunately, most indoor lighting systems do not approximate the same color spectrums as natural sunlight. Full-spectrum fluorescent lighting approximates the same spectrum as sunlight and has been shown to have positive effects on visual acuity and reduces hyperactivity and central nervous system fatigue. Incandescent lights favor the orange-red end of the spectrum, whereas fluorescent lighting emphasizes the yellow-green portion. It is important that the environment offer lighting options that can be controlled by the patient. The lighting source (where it is located in the room), intensity, and direction should be controllable by the patient.

Gardens and Paths

Access to natural light can be enhanced with window seating, access to an outdoor patio, or the use of gardens. The concept of healing gardens has become popular in the design of health care facilities. The intent of the gardens is to provide a relaxing retreat for patients and families who experience tremendous stress from their illness, treatment, and hospitalization.[11] The healing gardens incorporate fresh air, sunshine, quietness, and a green, growing environment. Often the garden is complete with a fish pond or a fountain for the sound effects of cascading water. Park benches are strategically located to allow small group interaction or solitude, depending on the patients' wishes. The healing gardens must provide both shade and sunny areas, be accessible to physically impaired persons, and include plants that are pleasing, colorful, and whose fragrance or blossoms are hypoallergenic. Labeled herb gardens can also provide a fragrance and taste experience for some patients. Inspiring sculptures, fountains, or religious statues can provide pleasant visual stimulation.

Akin to the concept of healing gardens, the use of walking paths within the healing garden or labyrinths has been considered to be therapeutic and relaxing. The labyrinths provide a pleasant area for cardiac rehabilitation patients to exercise and a place for staff to walk for relaxation. Researchers have indicated that the labyrinths often have spiritual symbolism and were used in many ancient cultures to promote healing.

Color

The use of color for healing is not new: early healers throughout history used color as a healing agent and to diagnose illness. Some believe that a body aura, vibrating light that surrounds and follows the body's contours, indicates the presence of illness or disease before physical pain is experienced. Specific colors in the spectrum are thought to affect certain parts of the body, mind, or emotion of the person, and the laying on of color can facilitate the healing of certain problems.[12]

Color in artwork, comfortable furnishings, or wall coverings can promote healing by allowing patients to relax, enjoy visual stimulation, or focus on art that simulates restful nature scenes.[13] Choosing the art must be done with sensitivity to culture, geographical area, interior color scheme, and the amount of light and nature views. The art itself might provide visual views of nature if the health center is in an urban setting. In darker rooms, a sunny, light-colored, bright picture can provide a sense of light. By adding carefully chosen artwork, it is possible to evoke emotion, create environments, and enhance healing. Areas that, in the minds of patients, family and staff, were in need of remodeling might even be renewed through art.

Furnishings

Furnishings should be durable, comfortable, and cheery. The furniture, accessories, artwork, and wall and floor coverings work together to create a pattern of color and visual interest. Together, they also give a subliminal message. Was the place designed with its clients in mind? Will clients relate to or enjoy the accessories in the space? Do personal mementos in the room make the area feel warm and welcoming? The addition of family photos and pictures of mothers and babies and women of all ages and stages of life provide a humanness to the room. Handiwork such as crochet, tapestries, quilts, needlepoint, or cross-stitch adds a "women's touch" to the space. Chairs and sofas should be plump, comfortable, inviting, and placed in ways that enhance social interaction or solitude and privacy.

In hospital settings, it is essential to include space and furniture for the family and to acknowledge that women are traditionally the center of most families. Even when ill or hospitalized, women are usually responsible for making plans for the families' meals, child care, or school schedules. The true family-centered approach to health care ensures that family members feel welcome in the environment. Furnishings should include comfortable seating for the visiting family and the option of a fold-down, fold-out bed arrangement if a family member chooses to stay as support. Making the family comfortable in the environment will create a feeling of well being for the patient.

Smells

Hospitals are known for their smells, and not necessarily pleasant ones. The combination of pharmaceuticals, chemical agents used for cleaning, disinfecting, and sterilizing, and food preparation smells create an environment that may not promote comfort.

Fragrances evoke memories of things past, and fragrances that suggest a homelike environment have been used to facilitate healing environments. Some hospitals and women's health centers use bowls of sachet, floral arrangements, green plants, and even cookies baking in an oven to convey a sense of home and relaxation. Aromatherapy has become very popular, and aromatherapy diffusers can also be used to promote feelings of rest, relaxation, and well-being.

Sounds

Health care settings are notoriously noisy. Footsteps in the hallway, staff conversations, televisions and radios, carts moving from room to room, clanging and banging of stainless steel instruments and equipment, and endless intercom announcements—all create anything but a healing environment. Unfortunately, outpatient settings are not much better. In this setting, the patient is subjected to phones and fax machines, staff conversations, televisions, and other mindless but noxious sounds. In planning healing health care settings, every possible way to reduce noise should be considered. Nurses, physicians, and other health care professionals can be supplied with nonaudible beepers to locate them so that the use of patient room intercoms or overhead speakers can be reduced. Hallways can be carpeted to reduce the noise level from carts, foot traffic, and communication.

Giving the patient earphones and the choice of relaxing music or videos (particularly relaxation tapes or videos on humorous subjects) can provide positive distraction and promote healing. The sound of water from a miniature fountain, birds singing, or other sounds in nature accompanied by soft classical music can be used in waiting areas to calm the anxious patient or family member.

Staff need to be sensitized to noise and look for every means to reduce it. When staff become aware of noise in their environment, they will begin to seek out more positive sounds as a substitute.

Privacy

All patients desire privacy. Because women are particularly sensitive to invasions of privacy, this criterion is especially significant to women's health center design—and the design can benefit everyone. Registration and admitting areas should ensure privacy as should triage and observation bays where a curtain wall often separates patients. A full-walled cubicle is the preferred design to ensure sound and visual privacy for the patient.

The angle of the bed in a room can facilitate privacy for the patient also. Unfortunately, many LDRs, LDRPs, and exam rooms are currently designed with the door facing the foot of the bed or exam table. An optimal design ensures that the foot of the bed or exam table points away from the door.

Patient dressing areas in exam rooms must be carefully considered to ensure patient privacy. Many consist of a corner of the room with a curtain that's neither wide enough nor heavy enough for a sense of privacy. Often the woman is not provided a private area to hang her under and outer clothing, making it embarrassing when the physician enters the room. A wall-mounted closet for storage of clothing can eliminate this problem. The inside of the closet door can be designed with a mirror and shelving for antiperspirant spray, hair spray, and fragrance samples for the woman's convenience after the exam.

Traditional exam rooms provide a paper examination gown and a paper lap drape for the examination. Neither provide privacy for the woman. Women's health centers should demonstrate sensitivity for the woman's privacy during exams and supply cloth coverlets for the examination table and possibly cloth gowns that have snap enclosures to facilitate patient examination. Some centers offer terry cloth or seersucker bathrobes for additional privacy, particularly if the patient is required to walk down the hall to the bathroom or lab for specimen collection before dressing.

Protection of the patient's privacy should be considered one of the most critical elements in a women's health center. The location and adjacency of certain areas should be critically analyzed, such as the admitting area and the lobby; the location of the weight scale and its adjacency to any public area; and the location of bathrooms or change areas with mammography or exam rooms. Privacy for the patients must be carefully guarded in the physical design and in all professional interactions with the patient.

A MULTITUDE OF HEALING ENVIRONMENTS

What constitutes a healing environment for women? A healing environment promotes a sense of wholeness for the woman and is sensitive to her unique needs for knowledge in self-care and the care of others for which she is responsible. The environment should foster a sense of caring, social support, and interconnectedness between provider and patient.

A healing environment for women provides a comprehensive array of programs that serve to improve her health, repair her body, and restore her mind and soul. To this end, any healing environment for women will include inpatient programs and services and outpatient screening and diagnostic programs to prevent illness and promote health. It will include an array of educational programs to empower women to participate in decision making regarding their own care and that of others in the family. Education will be presented in methods that call for the participation of women in their own learning. This might include books, pamphlets, audiovisual materials, Internet sites, and interactive group sessions. Support groups to facilitate social support for weight loss, infertility, menopause, and other related issues will ease healing of the mind and body.

Many women's facilities across the country are developing the concept of healing spas for women's centers. One example of this concept is at Scottsdale Health Care in Scottsdale, Arizona. The healing spa in the women's center will include a day spa for women, massage therapy, exercise therapy, and other integrative modalities. Other women's centers have collaborated with their centers for fitness and lifestyle management to provide "especially for women" programs at certain times of the day. During this time, women have the opportunity to avail themselves of exercise physiologists, personal trainers, water and massage therapy, tai chi, and other types of therapies.

A healing environment for women must include, or make available, behavioral health services. Educational programs, support programs, and actual therapeutic sessions provided by clinical psychologists, licensed clinical social workers, and marriage, family and child counselors can be most beneficial in supporting women through the various transitions of ages and stages of life.

SUMMARY

Health and healing connotes a sense of wholeness and prescribes the person's ability to act, react, and adapt to changes and challenges in the environment. To meet the women's market, providers must create physical as well as psychosocial environments that support the woman's need to be whole and complete in mind, body, emotion, and spirit.

Their design for healing environments must be intentional, sensitive, and based on the combined knowledge of a variety of fields, ranging from architecture to psychology.

Notes

1. Ulrich, R. S. "View Through a Window May Influence Recovery from Surgery." *Science,* 1984, *224,* 420–421.
2. Peplau, H. *Interpersonal Relations in Nursing.* New York: Putnam, 1952.
3. Levine, M. *Introduction to Clinical Nursing.* (2nd ed.) Philadelphia: Davis, 1973.
4. Nightingale, F. *Notes on Nursing.* Philadelphia: Lippincott, 1992.
5. Venolia, C. *Healing Environments.* Berkeley, Calif.: Celestial Arts, 1988.
6. Venolia, *Healing Environments,* p. 7.
7. Venolia, *Healing Environments,* p. 11.
8. Carlson, L. K. "Creating Designs That Heal." *California Hospitals,* May-June 1992, pp. 11–12.
9. "Research Identifies What Consumers Want." *Aesclepius,* 1998, *7*(2), 1.
10. Stichler, J. F., and Weiss, M. A. "Quality in Women's Health Services from the Perspective of the Patient, Nurse, Physician, and the Payor." Unpublished manuscript, 1998.
11. Marcus, C. C., and Barnes, M. "Therapeutic Benefits of Gardens in Health Care Facilities: An Evaluative Study and Design Recommendations." *Journal of Healthcare Design,* 1997, *8,* 23 29.
12. Stein, D. *All Women Are Healers.* Freedom, Calif.: Crossing Press, 1990.
13. Malkin, J. "Decor-Therapy." *San Diego Union-Tribune,* June 30, 1996, p. H-1; Mayberry, S. O., and Zagon, L. *The Power of Color: Creating Healthy Interior Spaces.* New York: Wiley, 1995.

CHAPTER SIXTEEN

Women's Health as a Strategic Initiative

Genie James
C. Ann Boeke

C. Ann Boeke, M.S., C.H.E., is a consultant in women's health services. She was previously director of Women's Ambulatory Initiatives at Mercy Health System in Philadelphia and director of corporate planning and development as well as executive director of the nationally acclaimed women's centers for Bellevue Women's Hospital in New York.

How does one develop a women's health strategy for a hospital or health system? The most critical step is identifying how a women's health initiative will fit into and supplement the organization's overall strategy for protecting or gaining market share and maximizing revenue streams. Remember that a women's health strategy means much more than reproductive medicine. Examine how women affect referrals, utilization, and provider selection, and women's health takes on a new dimension.

This chapter describes several ways to develop a focus on and commit resources to women's health, for no one solution fits every market.

One piece of good news: the reimbursement shifts that have forced an emphasis on ambulatory care have done women's health a favor. The rise of ambulatory care has supported more choices, more convenience, and more cost efficiency—features the female consumer has been demanding for decades. Today, providers must determine how best to make money by developing products and services around a philosophy that emphasizes health promotion, education, the creation of sensitive settings for service delivery, gender-based medicine, and a commitment to physical, psychosocial, and spiritual health.

The first step is to develop a strategic plan.

DEVELOPING A STRATEGIC PLAN FOR A WOMEN'S HEALTH INITIATIVE

The challenge for any provider searching for an appropriate women's health strategy is finding one that will synchronize with their organizational objectives and financial responsibilities. The provider's objectives for women's health services must align with the organization's critical strategic concerns. Providers must be very clear regarding both the internal and external forces that will affect—and ultimately drive—the success of any new venture (see Table 16.1). Local market strategies must be derived from the unique variables defining each opportunity. Some of those variables include the following:

- Managed care penetration
- Degree of provider integration
- Market share
- Current utilization patterns
- Competitive situation
- Geography
- Social and cultural variables

In addition, it is wise to consider your organization's current financial position and availability of resources.

All this requires a good bit of market research. Before proposing a model, check with customers to see if they would use it. The success of every new strategy plays out in the market. Ask your customers

External Forces	Internal Forces
Downsizing inpatient	Strengths and weaknesses
Expanding outpatient	Reputation
Closing hospitals, mergers, alliances	Location for accessibility
Systems and network development	Medical staff
Regulatory environment	Specialties services
Managed care	Current services that may contribute to
Competitive factors	your women's health center
Community health needs	Organizational culture; political
	environment

Table 16.1.   Developing a Strategic Plan.

what they want! This can be accomplished via customized surveys, focus groups, client surveys, patient profiles, and other customer feedback loops that may already be in place within the organization.

Be very sure to get past generalities and really know your customer. "Women" is much too broad. Get specific. The strategic planning process must drill down to the details for each of the following:

• Women: age groups, ethnic groups, socioeconomic groups

• Managed care organizations

• Community organizations

• Corporations and businesses

Your strategic plan will be derived from an analysis of the data gathered. It should begin with a mission statement that clarifies the intention of the women's health initiative, states what the initiative hopes to accomplish, and keeps everyone focused in the same direction. The mission statement should be followed by a vision statement defining the major functions of the initiative, the levels of care to be included, the programs, products, and services to be offered, the target population that should drive the business, and how the initiative will exist in relationship to the sponsoring organization. The strategic plan should then offer a framework for this vision. It is the road map that enables an organization to first buy into and then move aggressively toward a common goal.

DEFINING A MODEL THAT WILL WORK

Once you have data on internal and external market forces as well as consumer preferences and demand requirements, determine how you want to position your women's health model within your organization. How do you define the model that will work? Here are a few options.

Women's Health Center Without Walls

In a center without walls, services are dispersed throughout the hospital and are typically positioned from an educational and marketing point of view. This approach generally provides information, referral services, education, and some in-house diagnostic services such as mammography. Two factors that can position this as a model of choice are lack of resources (capital) or lack of senior management perspective regarding the import of women's health to the more profitable upstream referral services.

Women's Center with Walls

A center with walls moves a step further. Often it is within the hospital but set apart by both its encapsulated physical structure and its specialized function. Often it is a pavilion, wing, or unit. Anecdotal feedback indicates that, because it begins to clearly establish a unique identity, the medical and professional staff of this model begin the process of bonding more closely around a mission that is specific to women's health.

Comprehensive Ambulatory Center

The comprehensive ambulatory center makes a statement regarding a philosophy of gender-based medicine and a sensitivity to consumer demand for convenience and one-stop shopping. A comprehensive ambulatory center offers services beyond reproductive health. In addition to education and diagnostic services, it offers medical services and some form of case management.

Freestanding Women's Hospital

A freestanding women's hospital is a specialty-niche model. Some physician practice management organizations have begun to take this approach in an attempt to move beyond the narrow profit margins associated with managing OB/GYN practices and to capture some of the facility fee. This model is more likely to be seen in competitive marketplaces where a niche player is attempting to come in and corner a component of the market share or where a hospital or health system believes that a stand-alone facility dedicated to women's health will differentiate it in the marketplace. Two variables are key if this kind of approach is the one of choice: access to capital and physician buy-in.

Service Line Approach

With the advent of network development, continued industry consolidation, and systems growth, most experts expect that the service line approach will continue to grow in popularity. This approach is chosen many times because of its potential to maximize quality while minimizing cost. This is accomplished by integrating planning, marketing, and finance into product design and implementation. The characteristics cited as critical to survival and success include flexibility, strategic thinking, risk taking, and the ability to articulate the vision for the service line and to enroll others—over whom one might not have direct authority—in that vision. Instead of a single inpatient unit, the focus is on a bigger picture: a product line, the cost of providing health care to a population, managing enrollees, risk identification, and utilization management.[1]

CASE STUDIES: WOMEN'S HEALTH INITIATIVES

Today, both payors or employers and female consumers demand horizontal integration and full-spectrum coordination of care. Although obstetrics remains the most important clinical service to payors, inpatient care may not occur at all during the process of caring for a woman for a year of her life. A shift among health care organizations and physicians to a "covered life" mentality is critical to meet the needs of payors, employers, and female consumers alike.[2] How can you strategically position your women's health initiatives within your system of care? This section looks at a few organizations that have done just that.

NORTH IOWA MERCY HEALTH CENTER: A LIFE SPAN OF CARE

North Iowa Mercy Health Center's women's health strategy incorporates several models and demonstrates a commitment to developing a life span of care for women. The center's market research estimated that 2,200 women would be diagnosed and 590 would die of breast cancer in Iowa in 1995. Breast cancer incidence rates had increased about 2 percent each year since 1980, reaching 110 cases per 100,000 women. Still, despite increased incidence, the mortality rate for breast cancer had remained relatively stable. The trend toward a greater proportion of breast cancers being diagnosed at an early stage was viewed as promising and supportive of activities aimed at awareness and early detection such as education and outreach activities. Increased access and utilization of mammography and clinical breast exams are obtainable and measurable outcome data. Diagnosis of early-stage breast cancer allows the woman and her health care provider options in therapy. Treatment for early-stage breast cancer is also less costly—approximately $11,000 versus $143,000 for late stage. In addition to early detection and screening opportunities, the center recognized a need to provide education to women regarding treatment options. The existing system did not allow for a coordinated, multidisciplinary educational and treatment planning process. Consequently, the recommendation was made to address this need by developing a comprehensive ambulatory center, that is, a breast health center, utilizing a multidisciplinary team to review and recommend treatment as well as to provide a care management approach to patients.

A different approach was required for North Iowa Mercy Health Center to address two other objectives within its women's health strategic initiative. Those objectives were to reduce domestic violence against women and increase recognition of women's health as having a substantive impact on the delivery of care across the continuum throughout the North Iowa Mercy Health Network.

It was determined that the recommended strategies to address these objectives would not require new bricks and mortar. This time a center without walls was recommended. Some of the action steps involved education, collaboration across the community, and community awareness campaigns, including newsletters, resource guides, and targeted media relationships. It is important to note the characteristics that led to deciding on this approach. Neither domestic violence nor the establishment of a broader definition of women's health can be easily located under a single service line definition. Both involve the community at large and its inherent social structure and overall health status indicators. Consequently, it would be impossible for a provider system to take sole responsibility for addressing these concerns.

VANDERBILT UNIVERSITY: FREESTANDING WOMEN'S HOSPITAL

"Sometimes the old ways come around again," said Roxanne Spitzer, the Vanderbilt University professor who helped secure funding for a new birthing center in east Nashville. "It's the old way of delivery at home but with a much higher level of safety." It will look more like home than hospital, with living rooms and kitchens for the families, large bedrooms, and baths for delivery. The birthing center will employ nurse midwives to deliver babies in a more natural atmosphere than hospitals. Paid for by a $5.2 million

Kellogg Foundation grant, the facility will be the first freestanding birthing center in Nashville. Although the center will initially be operated by money provided in the grant, administrators plan for it to be run by the community within several years.[3]

SUTTER HEALTH SYSTEM: A SERVICE LINE APPROACH

Sutter Health System has committed resources to expand women's health services across its system. This integrated delivery approach to women's health includes twenty-six acute care hospitals, seven long-term care centers, outpatient care centers in more than one hundred northern California communities, and relationships with more than five thousand physicians. Shelly McGriff, assistant administrator for women's and children's services at five of the hospitals, reports several outcomes directly attributable to service line management. Overall, the implementation of service line management resulted in a 2 percent improvement in margins. Included in this are 4 percent savings in labor and delivery supply costs from standardizing packs, and additional savings from standardizing other supplies, forms, and educational materials. Moreover, when McGriff instituted systemwide service lines in the five hospitals, she noted both an improvement in management efficiency and a 10 percent decrease in the cost of management.[4]

SUMMARY

The case studies give a brief glimpse into how the hospitals or health systems defined models that work for them. Determining which one will work for you requires an understanding of local market dynamics, targeted data collection, primary market research, analytical thought, and the factoring in of all those subtle and sexy—or perhaps simply less obvious—variables like buy-in, politics, organizational culture, and commitment to a mission that ultimately define success.

There are no cookie-cutter solutions, but there are some common denominators between the models that are working at the local level. Obviously, the finances must work. Reimbursement is shrinking and providers intending to operate in the environment of the future must be prepared to take on risk-based arrangements, become accountable for the health of enrolled populations, figure out a feasible way to begin to emphasize health promotion and disease prevention, focus on ambulatory care, and determine how women's health really does fit into this new paradigm of care. Models of care that emphasize health promotion, education, sensitive settings for service delivery, gender-based medicine, and a commitment to psychosocial and spiritual health need to be evaluated to be sure they can indeed make money.

Those choosing a specific model of care should evaluate its value to their complete enterprise of health services delivery.

Notes

1. Graf, M. "The Service Line Director's Survival Guide." *Business Review of Women's Health and Reproductive Medicine,* Oct.-Dec. 1997, pp. 16–20.
2. Graf, "The Service Line Director's Survival Guide."
3. Yates, J. "Old-Fashioned Birthing Returns to East Nashville." *Nashville Tennessean,* Nov. 22, 1998, p. 1A.
4. Yates, J. "Old-Fashioned Birthing Returns to East Nashville."

CHAPTER SEVENTEEN

Medicare Risk

Evolution and Implications for Women

Kimberly Weiss

> *Kimberly Weiss is a consultant for BDC Advisors, LLC, a health care consulting firm in San Francisco. She formerly served as executive director of the National Association for Women's Health.*

This chapter examines the dynamics of managing the health of the Medicare population. Why focus on the Medicare patient when considering a women's health strategy? The statistics documenting the percentage of seniors in the marketplace and how many of those are women provides the answer. A gender-specific understanding of the senior market requires understanding the female patient and her utilization and access patterns. Women are already the majority of the Medicare market:

- 57 percent of all Medicare beneficiaries are women
- 63 percent of those seventy-five and over are women
- 72 percent of those eighty-five and over are women
- 68 percent of women experience chronic conditions, mostly in older age

As the women go through menopause, they will become susceptible to an increasing number of health problems—osteoporosis, depression, migraines, coronary heart disease, and urinary incontinence—conditions further complicated by the late age of disease onset.[1] With those numbers in hand, it is obvious the global female Medicare population will continue to demand health care services. It can be anticipated that the same phenomenon will occur in your market.

MEDICARE FOR THE ELDERLY: PAST AND PRESENT

Established in 1965, the Medicare program was designed to meet the medical care needs of the elderly in the United States. Today, the program is in danger of bankruptcy, and millions of elderly are in danger of growing old with no viable option for health insurance.

The payment methodologies of Medicare have undergone a number of significant changes, sending shock waves through the industry. Most recently, Congress approved sweeping legislation allowing managed care organizations and providers to offer risk-based Medicare. Payors, providers, and patients must now determine the most appropriate response to this legislation, much of which has not yet even been clearly articulated by Congress.

Medicare benefits are offered to both men and women, but it has particular significance to women and to those who provide care to women, for the following reasons:

- Women comprise over 57 percent of Medicare's enrollees
- Women experience more chronic conditions than men as they age, resulting in higher utilization rates
- Women have significantly lower incomes than men in older age, thus they have less income available for health care, relying even more on Medicare than men do.

History of the Medicare Program

Medicare was originally designed as a fee-for-service program. Persons age sixty-five and over who are entitled to Social Security are automatically eligible to participate in the Medicare program. Medicare consists of two primary parts, Part A and Part B. Part A benefits are generally provided automatically to persons age sixty-five and over and covers a portion of the beneficiary's inpatient care, some skilled nursing, home health under certain conditions, and hospice care. Part B is optional and requires beneficiaries who participate to pay a monthly premium. It covers certain physician services, durable medical equipment, ambulance services, and other benefits. Beneficiaries can also elect to purchase a medigap policy that covers many of the services not covered by Part A or Part B.

By the end of its first year of operation, Medicare enrollees totaled approximately 19.1 million. Today, there are approximately 38 million Medicare beneficiaries. Costs have grown with enrollment. In 1997, Medicare Part A benefits totaled $137.8 billion, an increase of 7.1 percent over the prior year. Total disbursements for Medicare in 1997 were $213.57 billion.[2]

Since its enactment, Medicare has been subject to numerous legislative and administrative changes. Under the original Medicare legislation, payment to providers was made on a "reasonable cost" basis. However, after fifteen years, the federal government realized it would be unable to control skyrocketing costs under this system. In 1983, in an effort to control costs, the government established a new payment system for Medicare. Medicare payments, although still made on a fee-for-service basis, were altered to bring the system under control, and providers were paid under a plan known as the prospective payment system (PPS). Under PPS, diagnostic related groups (DRGs) were established to describe all inpatient events. "Values" were placed on the services related to treatment for each DRG. This predetermined value, a prospective payment, was made to hospitals for DRG services, as provided. Under PPS, providers gave the patient whatever care was necessary within that inpatient stay as it related to the noted DRG for the one prospective payment. The incentives were such that it was advantageous to provide more care rather than less, and costs continued to skyrocket. The Health Care Finance Administration (HCFA), which administers the Medicare program, continues to pay in this way for services provided to the beneficiary enrolled in the traditional Medicare plan.

A separate system has been used to pay for physician services. Prior to 1992, physicians were paid on a basis of "reasonable charge" (defined in various ways). As with hospitals, physicians who accepted Medicare payments under this system were motivated to provide more, not fewer, services to their patients. The Government responded to rising costs by changing the reimbursement system. Starting in January 1992, allowed charges were redefined as the lesser of the submitted charges or a fee schedule based on a resource-based relative value scale (RBRVS). The intention was to bring costs under control by matching payment to the relative amount of resources expended for services provided.

The changes to Medicare reimbursement approved in 1983 and 1992 shocked the industry, but the Balanced Budget Act of 1997 (BBA), which legislated Medicare risk, will have an even greater effect than those two previous changes combined. BBA created Medicare Part C, authorizing the Medicare + Choice (M + C) program and other reforms. It calls for the largest Medicare cuts in the program's history, $116.4 billion over five years. BBA will have a profound effect on providers, health plans, and Medicare beneficiaries. Congress has lofty goals for BBA. It is designed to increase choice for beneficiaries, promote competition, increase efficiencies, and bring high-quality care to an increasing number of elderly in the most efficient manner.

Medicare Risk Programs

In 1985, Medicare risk programs were born with the signing of the Tax Equity and Fiscal Responsibility Act (TEFRA). TEFRA established demonstration projects to determine the feasibility, advantages, and risks of offering Medicare beneficiaries a managed care option. Health plans participating in Medicare risk received monthly per member per month rates set at approximately 95 percent of the average expenses for fee-for-service beneficiaries in a given county (95 percent of AAPCC rates). Over five years, the performance of the Medicare HMO demonstration projects was measured, and the results were favorable. By 1992 over 1.2 million Americans were participating in Medicare HMOs. Managed care companies, through their contracts with providers, were able to provide care to Medicare beneficiaries at reduced costs while maintaining patient satisfaction. Managed care, therefore, could potentially provide the much-needed solution to escalating costs.

In 1986, Medicare risk enrollment was 0.8 million. Growth has been unprecedented. Currently, of the approximately 38 million Medicare beneficiaries, 6.5 million (17 percent) have joined managed care plans. Between 1993 and 1996, enrollment grew by 33 percent annually and Medicare risk penetration rose from 3.4 percent to 28.1

percent. Commercial managed care took nearly a decade to capture 28 percent of the market.[3] Geographic expansion has also been extensive, with substantive coverage in states across the country.

The federal government expects continued growth in Medicare managed care enrollment, projecting a tripling of enrollment over the next ten years. Congressional assumptions place the overall number of Medicare managed care enrollees at approximately 25 percent of all beneficiaries by 2002 and 35 percent by 2007.

Increasing Beneficiaries' Choice

BBA's M + C program provides Medicare beneficiaries with a wider range of health plan choices. If the market responds to the BBA as the government predicted when it passed the legislation, Medicare beneficiaries will be able to choose to receive their benefits through a variety of options, beyond the traditional government-sponsored option. Choices will include the following:

• Health maintenance organizations (HMOs) with or without a point of service option

• Preferred provider organizations (PPOs)

• Provider service organizations (PSOs)

• Private fee-for-service payment arrangements

• Medical savings accounts (MSAs)

HMO and PPO Medicare risk plans operate as prepaid capitated arrangements under which incentives are reversed from those found with traditional fee-for-service Medicare. With Medicare risk, providers have an incentive to manage utilization rather than to maximize it.

HMOs AND PPOs   Point of service (POS) HMO products allow enrollees to self-refer to providers outside the primary network, usually for an added cost. They offer favorable pricing for in-network benefit utilization, require preauthorization for high-cost, out-of-network services, and require out-of-pocket co-pays. POS products offer the best of both worlds, access and choice, to enrollees. They are favorable transitional products for seniors who are reluctant to participate in managed care programs. However, because of the decreased level of control inherent in a POS program, delivery systems interested in participating in POS products must be relatively sophisticated in their ability to manage care. Those systems with highly sophisticated information and medical management systems, a large provider network, and the potential to establish appropriate cost-sharing structures are the most likely to succeed in this area. Sufficient management systems will ensure lower costs, whereas an extensive network will decrease the likelihood of out-of-network use. Cost-sharing structures that motivate beneficiaries to use in-network providers help to minimize out-of-network costs.

PSOs The Balanced Budget Act is designed to increase competition by encouraging the development of a larger variety of products and by increasing the number of companies offering these products. Built into the legislation are terms that will reduce the providers' barriers to entry into the managed care market. Restrictions related to the formation of provider services organizations have been loosened. PSOs are managed care contracting and delivery organizations that accept full risk for beneficiary lives.

Whereas Medicare + Choice organizations are required to be licensed by the state as a risk-bearing entity eligible to offer health insurance, the BBA allows a PSO to obtain a federal waiver if it meets certain criteria (such as the state failing to complete action on a licensing application within ninety days; denying the licensing application based on discriminatory treatment; or denying the licensing application based on the organization's failure to meet solvency requirements). In addition, minimum enrollment requirements are less than those required for other Medicare + Choice organizations; for PSOs, the enrollment requirement is 1,500 members in nonrural areas, 500 in rural areas (non-PSO Medicare risk plans are required to enroll 5,000 members in nonrural areas and 1,500 in rural areas). The BBA has eliminated the fifty-fifty rule that had required at least 50 percent non-Medicare enrollment in point-of-service plans.

Under the Balanced Budget Act, a PSO must be organized and operated by a health care provider or group of health care providers and must deliver at least 70 percent of services required by Medicare law; the remainder may come from contracts with other providers. The providers must have at least 51 percent financial interest in the PSO organization.

PSOs offer control over the premium, allowing providers the opportunity to maximize profit from Medicare risk. By engaging providers as managers and owners of health care delivery systems, it may be possible to reach the next level of cost savings while enhancing quality of care. Providers achieve Medicare risk savings by reducing hospital utilization through population and patient management strategies such as the implementation of clinical protocols, care management, wellness programs, and targeted intervention programs for health status improvement within the covered population.

PRIVATE FEE-FOR-SERVICE ARRANGEMENTS   A provision of BBA allows providers who opt out of the Medicare program to enter into private contracts with Medicare beneficiaries for Medicare-covered health services. These plans are not bound by Medicare rates and, therefore, providers may be paid at higher rates, increasing costs to beneficiaries who choose this option. The provider must agree not to submit any claims to Medicare within two years of signing a contract with a patient.[4] The law does not affect services not covered by Medicare. Physicians who provide Medicare enrollees with services not covered by Medicare may continue to charge Medicare enrollees for these services as they have always done and can also continue to participate in the Medicare program. To date, this option has been utilized rarely.

MEDICAL SAVINGS ACCOUNTS   The Balanced Budget Act also authorizes a medical savings account national demonstration project. Limited to 390,000 beneficiaries who enroll between January 1, 1999, and January 1, 2003, the program will allow participants to purchase a catastrophic health plan with deductibles and out-of-pocket expenses of not more than $6,000 in 1999. Beneficiaries will choose a health insurance policy to provide the coverage. The policy will determine the choice of doctors and benefits available. Medicare pays the insurance company a monthly premium for the beneficiary's coverage. If the premium for the plan is less than the Medicare + Choice capitation rate, the difference is deposited by the HCFA into the individual's MSA. The beneficiary pays for the cost of care until reaching the $6,000 deductible. At that point, the insurance company pays for some or all of the beneficiary's medical costs, depending on the plan. Interest in the MSA program thus far has been limited. Many experts question its long-term viability.

Beyond Medicare + Choice

In addition to establishing M + C, the BBA reduced fee-for-service payments to all providers. Projected cumulative average payment reductions for inpatient and outpatient services ranges from 5.6 percent in 1998 to 11.7 percent in 2002.[5] Medicare Part C also creates a new payment model designed to reduce disparities in rates across the country and to replace unpredictable fluctuations in the individual county rates with a more predictable national update factor. This revision in the law is designed to narrow the amount of payment variation across the country and to increase incentives for plans to operate in diverse geographic areas. The environment will increasingly be characterized by lower payments and greater cost control incentives. Little will remain of cost-based payment mechanisms by the year 2002; careful analysis of cost structures and operating expenses over the long term are essential.

Finding the Reductions

The single largest savings to result from BBA will come from reductions in the hospital inpatient prospective payment system inflation update factors through 2002. Under BBA, the rates of increase in PPS payments to hospitals are reduced to market basket minus 1.9 percent in 1999, market basket minus 1.8 percent in 2000 and market basket minus 1.1 percent in 2001. The rationale behind these reductions in the rates of increase stems from findings reported by the Prospective Payment Assessment Commission (ProPAC). Although hospitals and delivery systems disagree with its conclusions, ProPAC used hospital reporting data and found that high profit levels were being made on the PPS. In addition, the BBA mandated the following:

- Reductions in inpatient PPS capital payments to a 90-percent-of-cost factor.

- Reductions in disproportionate share payments; hospitals will calculate their DSH amounts and then reduce them by 2 percent in 1999 and an additional percentage point for each of the following three years.

- Payments for medical education must be carved out of the average adjusted per capita cost (AAPCC) rates over the next four years and be paid directly to the teaching hospitals, with incentives to reduce the numbers of residents

- Changes to and reductions in the physician RBRVS fee schedules

- An increase in payment for PAs, NPs, and CNSs from HCFA to 80 percent of the lesser of either the actual charge or 85 percent of the physician fee schedule amount.

• A new Outpatient Department Prospective Payment System for hospital outpatient department services. A fee schedule for all covered outpatient services will be developed.[6]

Payments Under Medicare Risk

The legislation is written such that risk payments to health plans will be based on the highest of the following:

• A blended rate, comprised of local and national AAPCC amounts

• A floor amount increased each year by the national per capita Medicare + Choice growth percentage

• A minimum 2 percent increase over the previous year.

On top of these moving parts, the BBA mandates budget neutrality so total payments under the new system must equal what total payments would have been if payment were based on the former county rates. Blended rates were not applied in 1998 and 1999 because, once the budget neutrality was applied, the blended rates were decreased by HCFA so significantly that they were no longer the highest of the three payment options.

County-specific payments will evolve over time. The ratio of the county to national average costs is being phased in such that the national average cost becomes a larger influence on the value of the ratio, rising to a fifty-fifty mix of local and national rates by 2002. At this point, HCFA predicts that counties in rural and other low-cost areas will see a significant increase in their payment rates.

No risk adjustment factor for enrollee health status has yet been added to the calculation of the capitated payment; however, by no later than March 1, 1999, a method of risk adjustment was to have been reported by HCFA to Congress. The adjustment would account for variations in per capita costs based on health status. It will also increase the incentive to enroll beneficiaries with serious health problems who may be able to benefit from care coordination. The data used to determine the risk adjustment calculation will be produced by the plans. As plans improve their capacity to produce accurate data, the risk adjustments will become more sensitive. Over the long term, HCFA expects to apply risk to outpatient care and nonhospitalized chronic care.

As with commercial managed care, under Medicare risk-based arrangements, profitability will be determined by the extent to which payors and providers can manage the costs of providing care. Health plans and providers are therefore challenged to build administrative, operational, and care management capabilities to manage utilization and ensure profitability.

THE FUTURE OF MEDICARE RISK

Recent widespread press has led some to question the viability of Medicare risk. A few of the headlines in 1998 read: "Medica Health Plan Pulls Its Medicare HMO from Four Minnesota Counties: 100,000 Forced to Find Other Coverage," "Health Plans Are Withdrawing from 300 Counties in 18 States," and "Governor of Florida Sues Health Plans for Withdrawing Medicare Risk Coverage."[7]

However, numerous health plans remain, demonstrating the likelihood of continued growth. Nationally, three-fourths of Medicare beneficiaries have a choice of at least one managed care plan, and more than half have a choice of two or more. Despite loud and negative press regarding Medicare managed care plans' ability to offer a managed care option to beneficiaries, for 1999 only 45,000 Medicare beneficiaries (less than 1 percent of the beneficiaries enrolled in managed care) will be left with no managed care options because of plan nonrenewals. As of October 13, 1998, forty-three HMOs operating under risk contracts were not renewing their contract, affecting only 221,000 beneficiaries, or 3.4 percent; all still have a choice for continued managed care coverage.[8]

Also, as of September 28, 1998, HCFA had forty-eight applications pending for new Medicare + Choice contracts and twenty-five pending applications for service area expansions from existing risk contractors, mostly for HMO-type coordinated care. Four applications are pending from PSOs. There was only one PPO application and no MSA or private fee-for-service plan applications.[9] So far, Medicare risk has survived.

Quality in Medicare Managed Care

The BBA includes important quality provisions for Medicare + Choice, requiring most plans to not only monitor quality but to improve it. All Medicare + Choice plans must report objective, standardized measurements of how well they provide care and services. They will use the Medicare Health Plan Employer Data and Information Set (HEDIS) to quantify performance. HEDIS measures eight components, including effectiveness of care (including functional status for enrollees over sixty-five); access and availability of care; satisfaction with the experience of care; health plan stability; use of services; cost of care; informed health care choices; and health plan descriptive information. Since January 1997, all Medicare approved plans have been required to submit Medicare HEDIS data.[10]

Beneficiary satisfaction with plan care and service will be measured using the Consumer Assessment of Health Plans Survey (CAHPS). CAHPS is a new survey tool released by the Department of Health and Human Services in February 1998 that will enable consumers to rate their health plans. HCFA plans to make the ratings public, allowing beneficiaries to use the survey information in choosing among plans. Competition based on quality will be promoted. It has also encouraged a reexamination by HCFA of the quality requirements in traditional FFS Medicare: "We are actively working to incorporate quality assessment and improvement into traditional fee-for-service Medicare . . . so beneficiaries will be able to make truly informed choices about all their options."[11]

Providers and delivery systems are ultimately accountable for the plans' ability to meet these requirements—and to succeed in doing so. A thorough understanding of these measures and a focus on ensuring satisfactory performance is critical.

THE INFLUENCE OF THE CONSUMER

Consumerism will strongly influence the evolution of the Medicare market. Money-back guarantees, no-waiting-in-line policies, and no-questions-asked returns are all expectations we readily apply in the retail market. However, customer service is rarely emphasized in health care. That may change. In the year 2001, there will be eighty million Americans over the age of fifty and they will consume about 70 percent of health care services. The future of health care in America will be dominated by how we learn to respond to and manage this vast population of seniors with multiple chronic conditions.[12]

Medicare provides over 35 percent of the annual revenue of many providers. Whether a delivery system chooses to participate in Medicare risk or not, strategies to position in the changing market will be necessary. Any provider interested in capturing the senior market, whether it be through risk contracts or Medicare fee-for-service, will only successfully compete if they demonstrate added value to their senior population. With an increase in competition in the Medicare market, seniors will begin to expect and plans will provide higher-quality service (phone calls returned, appointment times available). The bar is being raised; it will not be acceptable to provide Medicare managed care products with less than "fee-for-service service."

One particularly unique and intriguing aspect of Medicare risk is its retail-like characteristics. Medicare risk products are sold directly to seniors, one member at a time. Seniors who join Medicare risk plans will evaluate and compare the various products available to them, weighing the costs and benefits of each option. Because they have the opportunity to do so and know it might make a difference, seniors are beginning to define for themselves what they want from their health care providers. Products will be differentiated by their price and their features, much as are other types of retail products, such as clothing, cars, and food.

Thus providers interested in attracting the senior market must be in touch with their customers. Not surprisingly, seniors do not define quality in the same way that providers and plans have done. Seniors, especially female seniors, identify quality in relational terms. They care about whether they perceive that the doctor listened, whether the receptionist seemed to care, whether the hospital staff helped them find their way. The older female health care consumer measures quality by the quality of the experience. The dignity, care, and respect they receive may even outweigh clinical outcomes for them.[13] Prudent providers and health plans will understand and meet the service needs of the aging population and the soon-to-be-Medicare recipients, the baby boomers (who grew up with Nordstrom and Federal Express as benchmark service providers). Every encounter an elderly person has with a provider or a health plan should be a positive experience; if it is not, it may be a customer lost.

A critical success factor is the branding of services as senior-friendly. Such branding will require an understanding of your market's demand for and utilization of services. It will be important to bring services to seniors that they view as valuable. Because women comprise at least 57 percent of the Medicare market, market research—always important to understanding the needs of the market—must now be gender based. Providers that understand the female senior's needs as different from the male senior's needs will be more effective at capturing the market.

PARTICIPATION IN THE RISK MARKETPLACE

Providers who choose not to accept Medicare risk will be affected by the decreased increases in PPS payments, by the changes to reimbursement of hospital outpatient facilities, and by the changes in payments in medical education as well as other important changes resulting from the BBA. Managing cost and maintaining as many of the nonrisk seniors as possible through cost accounting and branding strategies, respectively, will help.

However, if the government's projections are correct and Medicare risk enrollment continues to grow at its current unparalleled rate, many providers are going to be forced to develop strategies to capture the Medicare risk market. Even in rural markets where the capitated payments are currently relatively low, capturing the market today in anticipation of increased rates in rural areas (as a result of the BBA) may be the best strategy.

Entering Medicare Risk

Although reimbursement for Medicare risk may seem low, providers that can master the art of managing the senior population and reducing the costs of serving that market will increase market share. How then to capture that market? Is it better to build capabilities by developing a PSO or to develop one or more alliances or contracts with managed care organizations?

To develop an answer, providers must explore market conditions. One key variable in decision making is provider indispensability, which is inversely proportional to the number of substitutes for the provider's services available in the market. A provider's indispensability will drive payor-provider alliance strategies.[14] "Indispensable" providers will have sufficient leverage over payors to negotiate favorable relationships or to develop their own contracting capabilities. Both market responses will drive an increase in alliances with payors. In markets where provider indispensability is low, however, nonexclusive all-payor contracting is more likely. In such instances, competition will lead to more competitive pricing and the elimination of supplemental premiums and expanded benefits.

Exclusivity

Some providers have chosen the strategy of developing exclusive or semiexclusive contracts with health plans to enter the Medicare risk market. Under such agreements, providers agree to share risk in exchange for a level of exclusivity. Unless the provider has substantial leverage over the payor in this relationship, providers will have to accept lower rates in exchange for exclusivity. Additionally, the indirect cost of accepting exclusive relationships is the cost of not being able to treat patients who are members of other payor's risk plans. Therefore, careful consideration must be given to the value of the number of lives gained versus the loss associated with the lives of beneficiaries who might choose another risk plan in which you are unable to participate.

Considering a PSO Strategy

Providers considering developing their own provider service organizations need to carefully consider a number of important questions. The investment required to build a PSO is significant; so is the risk. The decision to build a PSO can be made based on the answer to key strategic questions described here.

Do the economics make sense? Are there opportunities to reduce costs? Hospital care offers the largest opportunity to reduce costs. According to HCFA, the health care cost elements of the Medicare population are broken down as follows: 55 percent hospital; 15 percent primary care; 30 percent specialist care. "Best-in-class" Medicare risk programs have reduced inpatient utilization to 60 percent below Medicare fee-for-service averages.

Are the Medicare risk rates relatively high? In 1998, a new floor of $367 per member per month was established. HCFA predicts that its revised method of calculating reimbursement rates, further modified by its risk adjustment factor, will create increased incentives for risk coverage of Medicare beneficiaries in rural areas.

What is the nature of the market? Are there a sufficient number of the "right" seniors? Mount Carmel in Ohio recently encountered success by targeting seniors with medigap policies. It sold a Medicare risk product that offered all the benefits of medigap without the additional premium. Before entering a business relationship in which providers accept accountability for marketing the product, the market's senior population should be critically examined and segmented to ensure the interest in Medicare risk is sufficiently large.

Are there a sufficient number of physicians that will accept risk with you? According to the Health Care Advisory Board, over time, as the market matures, seniors entering Medicare risk care more about access to preferred doctors and hospitals. Therefore, a key to being able to market a Medicare risk product over the long term is a strong physician network. The retail nature of Medicare risk, however, also reduces the need for the broad coverage that is necessary in the commercial marketplace, allowing for success with smaller provider networks.

What does the payor market look like? Has managed care penetrated the market to a sufficient extent that the public is willing to join managed care contracts? If not, marketing may be substantially more difficult. The latest InterStudy's Competitive Edge 7.2 found that markets where HMOs are most established as commercial plans are also markets in which Medicare plans have been likely to grow.

Are you indispensable enough to payors that you rely on for other contracts that your entry into the managed care market will not lead to an unfavorable reaction on their part? Is there room in the market for another Medicare risk player? What percentage of the senior market has joined other plans? Voluntary Medicare risk disenrollment to date is low. Converting seniors from traditional Medicare is more easily accomplished than conversion from other Medicare risk products. Additionally, seniors who do not convert early when plans first enter the market are likely to expect a more extensive network and benefits.

Are you able to meet the regulatory requirements? Do you have the capability to manage administrative and operational efficiencies? Those who choose to accept Medicare risk will need to implement care management and operational strategies that account for decreased utilization, both in admissions and length of stay as well as decreased reimbursement for services.

The retail nature of Medicare risk provides a distinct opportunity to providers. Health care providers are generally more credible and trustworthy than managed care plans in the eyes of consumers. Mount Carmel, an integrated delivery system in Columbus, Ohio, recently learned through focus groups and other market research that Medicare beneficiaries are twice as likely to enroll in a managed care plan sponsored by a hospital than one developed by a health plan.[15] Therefore, providers that leverage their brand and capabilities, whether it be through a PSO or with a health plan, will be able to retain more of this important market.

Women's Health and Medicare Risk

Success in the Medicare risk market will depend on the extent to which the health care needs and utilization patterns of senior women are understood. Delivery systems, therefore, should conduct strategic analyses of their population, conduct gender sorts on their Medicare risk population, and use the gender-based knowledge of their population as a foundation for population management and program development strategies. Customer needs assessments should be conducted with a focus on gender differences. Highly targeted risk-focused demand and disease management strategies can then be developed. Physician education can be improved. Marketing and sales strategies can be carefully tailored to attract the female market. Costs can be reduced through directed efforts and the development of care management protocols aimed at conditions that affect the senior woman.

Despite the cries of woe from some women's groups that claim Medicare risk encourages cost cutting and decreases choice, Medicare risk offers many positive attributes to the elderly female consumer.

AFFORDABILITY   In 1996, 63 percent of the existing Medicare managed care plans offered zero premium options.[16] The majority of elderly women are on fixed incomes that limit their ability to afford even the most basic of the Medicare options. The average single woman over sixty-five years old earns under $20,000 per year. Medicare risk plans offer affordable, more predictable options.[17]

INCREASED COVERAGE   Medicare risk plans also offer richer benefits packages than traditional Medicare. Most Medicare risk plans cover services that are not covered at all or are covered with strict limits by traditional Medicare. Such benefits include routine physicals, mammograms, full hospitalization, one hundred days of skilled nursing facility care, and home care. Over half of them offer pharmacy benefits.

PREVENTION   As of January 1, 1998, Medicare covers a Pap smear and pelvic exam once every three years for all female Medicare beneficiaries (annually for women who are at high risk for cervical or vaginal cancer). Starting July 1, 1998, Medicare also expanded coverage of preventive benefits for beneficiaries at risk for osteoporosis and other bone abnormalities. Eligible beneficiaries will be able to have their bone mass measured once every two years. Although many advocates suggest that coverage for these preventive measures is not enough, relative to Medicare fee-for-service it is a substantial improvement. Market dynamics also suggest that benefits will improve as the market matures and competition increases, implying that coverage for these preventive measures are likely to increase if the market demands it.

CHOICE   The Balanced Budget Act increases a beneficiary's choice. Prior to the BBA, choices were extremely limited. Today, most Medicare eligibles can choose between an HMO, PPO, and traditional services. Depending on her needs, this type of market choice is highly desirable for an elderly woman.

INFORMATION   The Health Care Finance Administration has built strict marketing restrictions into Medicare + Choice. It mandates that plans provide accurate, timely information to all beneficiaries. In addition, it has developed a comprehensive nationwide education campaign to ensure that all Medicare eligibles understand their choices. Senior women today have more of an opportunity to understand their health care insurance options than ever before.

QUALITY   Seniors in Medicare risk plans to date are satisfied with their plans. Voluntary disenrollment is low and those who do disenroll are likely to reenroll in another risk plan.[18] According to the American Hospital Association, seniors in Medicare managed care plans are more satisfied with their plan than are seniors in FFS Medicare.

KNOWLEDGE   HCFA's mandate that plans measure quality along similar attributes and its plan to publish the results of those quality measures will allow Medicare beneficiaries to make more informed choices.

DECREASING SELECTION BIAS   Richard Smith, vice president for policy and research at the American Association of Health Plans, claims that the potential for selection bias with Medicare risk will disappear as more seniors enroll in risk plans. Some suggest the selection bias is only minimal. For example, the August 19, 1996, issue of *Modern Healthcare* published the results of a Price Waterhouse study that found few differences in the health status between HMO enrollees and the fee-for-service population.

COMPETITION   Increased competition is generally good for the consumer. Existing health plans will most likely respond to the threat of increased competition and PSO development by adding value and decreasing prices. In the long run, innovation will be the result. Product innovation and alliances between health plans and payors could very well be a superior health product for tomorrow's senior.

Health plans are likely to incorporate what they have learned about women's health in the commercial market into their Medicare risk plans. Recognizing the role that women play in the health care market, the American Association of Health Plans has acknowledged plans that provide exemplary services to women. Recently published monographs on exemplary women's health programs offered through health plans in the United States outlined common themes among those that are striving to meet women's needs, including the following:[19]

• Cultivating provider input in the design phase of any project

• Multidisciplinary committees to address women's health issues

• Benchmarks and evaluation programs to gauge success

• Linkages and partnerships with local community-based organizations

• A conscious effort to drive significant change in the culture and practice patterns of the traditional biomedical model

In the long term, Medicare risk is expected to mirror the commercial risk market. Overall, commercial HMO members "have lower hospital admission rates, shorter hospital length of stay, the same or more primary care physician visits per enrollee, less use of expensive procedures and tests and greater use of preventive services."[20] HMO members rate their overall satisfaction with their health plans higher than people in indemnity plans. If Medicare risk options evolve in a similar fashion as the commercial HMOs, elderly women are likely to benefit substantially from Medicare risk.

SUMMARY

Given the economics and rapid changes in the environment, provider and payor organizations should develop strategies to obtain the Medicare risk market and to manage that market by focusing on elderly female customers, monitoring their needs, utilization, and purchasing behaviors closely.

The right provider strategy will depend on timing, environmental factors, and the organization's structure and current strategy. For sustainable competitive advantage, providers should ask the following questions on a regular basis:

- Who are the seniors in my market and what do they need and expect?
- Who is currently meeting those needs?
- What are my competitors doing and what are their strengths?
- What are the AAPCC rates?
- Can I provide services within those rates?
- What value and products can I produce and bring to the market without alliances?
- Should I go it alone or should I develop alliances with others?
- How will those I choose not to develop alliances with respond?
- Can I afford that response? If not, how do I change the response?

Although delivery systems have control over or influence most of the answers to these questions, they have no influence over the first question: Who are the seniors in my market and what do they need and expect? Yet the success of the entire strategy depends on the answer to this question. The characteristics of senior markets across the country vary, yet they all have one thing in common—they are mostly women. Women are driving the Medicare risk market. Therefore, providers and payors who have developed the infrastructure and network to enter the risk market can obtain a competitive advantage by gaining a thorough gender-specific understanding of the senior market and by developing strategies grounded in the understanding that the female population drives the costs and the revenue in the Medicare marketplace.

Notes

1. "Explosive Growth in the Demand for Women's Health Services Is Examined in a Report Published by Decision Resources." *PR Newswire,* Apr. 30, 1997.

2. Health Care Finance Administration.

3. *Medicare Strategy: The Race to Retail Coverage.* Washington, D.C.: Health Care Advisory Board, 1997.

4. Gottlich, V. *Summary of the New Medicare + Choice Program.* Washington, D.C.: National Senior Citizens Law Center, 1998.

5. BDC Advisors, health care consultants, San Francisco.

6. *The Balanced Budget Act of 1997: Medicare and Medicaid Changes.* Wilton, Conn.: Deloitte & Touche, 1997.

7. *Minneapolis Star,* Sept. 30, 1998; American Association of Health Plans press release, Oct. 5, 1998; *New York Times,* Oct. 17, 1998.

8. Health Care Finance Administration. "Protecting Medicare Beneficiaries After HMOs Withdraw." Washington, D.C.: Health Care Finance Administration, Oct. 13, 1998.

9. Michael Hash, deputy administrator of the Health Care Financing Administration. Testimony to the House Commerce Subcommittee on Health. Oct. 2, 1998.

10. Bruce Merlin Fried, director of the Office of Managed Care, Health Care Finance Administration. Statement to the Senate Committee on Labor and Human Resources. Mar. 6, 1997.

11. Fried statement.

12. Clark, B. "Older, Sicker, Smarter and Redefining Quality: The Older Consumer's Quest for Patient-Driven Service." *Healthcare Forum Journal,* Jan.-Feb. 1998.

13. Clark, "Older, Sicker."

14. BDC Advisors.

15. "Integrated Healthcare Report." *Healthcare Megatrends,* Jan. 1998.

16. Gottlich, *Summary.*

17. U.S. Census Bureau.

18. *HCFA Disenrollment Rates Report.* 1995.

19. *Advancing Women's Health: Health Plans' Innovative Programs in Breast Cancer.* Washington, D.C.: American Association of Health Plans, 1998.

20. Bernstein, A. "Women's Health in HMOs: What We Know and What We Need to Find Out." *Women's Health Issues,* Feb. 1996, 6(1).

CHAPTER EIGHTEEN

Relationship-Centered Care
Hope on the Horizon

Genie James

D oes managed care work? Not yet; it hasn't really been tried. The industry is still reeling from the impact of changing reimbursements. Providers are not actually managing care, but simply trying to manage cost.

Providers committed to differentiating themselves in the marketplace while also fulfilling mission statements that speak of their oath as healers are standing between two realities. The business reality is that you have to do more with less and in less time. This does not lend itself to what some may call a touchy-feely approach to the delivery of care. The other reality is that the consumer is rebelling at the mechanization of a healing industry. Is it possible to stay in business and also deliver health care services in a personalized and caring environment?

Providers that find a way to commit to a relationship-centered approach to service delivery are reminders that health care begins with an intimate one-on-one interaction. Pain is personal. Family members or friends who are sick, hurting, or at risk are fundamental realities. Those in the industry—the business—of health care must remember that true care is not a matter of utilization tracking reports or reports of revenue and market share. The winners will see their rewards in the faces of their patients. And if they successfully integrate their mission with their business strategies, they should ultimately realize their rewards in long-term financial and operational viability.

There are dozens of such winners; following are descriptions of a few. They fall under familiar headings: advocacy, outreach, family-centered care, and holistic health.

ADVOCACY

An advocate is one who champions a cause for another, in this case one who champions the cause of a patient. Bringing the patient into the care dynamic is one of the most essential tenets of a relationship-centered approach to health care.

The National Breast Cancer Coalition (NBCC) began in May of 1991. NBCC's goals are to increase research into the cause, treatment, and cure for breast cancer; to improve access for all women to high-quality breast cancer screening, diagnosis and treatment; and to increase the influence of breast cancer survivors in research, clinical trials, and national policy.

Since its founding, NBCC has helped increase federal funding for breast cancer research more than fivefold, from $90 million to more than $500 million, and has brought the issue to the office of the President of the United States and the halls of Congress and state legislatures. NBCC conceived and continues to be the driving force behind the National Action Plan on Breast Cancer, perhaps the most important comprehensive and integrated national strategy to end breast cancer. NBCC's successes are possible because it has built a nationwide network of grassroots advocates, including local hospitals, physicians, and care givers committed to advancing public policy that will lead to the eradication of breast cancer.

"The Face of Breast Cancer: A Photographic Essay" is one vehicle for ensuring that breast cancer remains at the forefront of the nation's agenda. It is an exhibit that was funded when the health care industry realized that education and awareness are key components of an aggressive marketing strategy. Created through a gift from Bristol-Meyers Squibb Oncology, it is a project of the National Breast Cancer Coalition Fund. All donations are tax-deductible.[1]

The exhibit humanizes the statistics and helps viewers grasp the epidemic proportions of the disease by focusing on individual women behind the numbers. It is a reminder that although we must speak out about the fact that forty-six thousand women die of breast cancer each year, these women are not mere numbers. They were mothers, wives, partners, friends.

The sixty-two women in the original exhibit represent every state. They reflect the diverse ages, ethnic backgrounds, professional lives, and life styles of those diagnosed with breast cancer. They represent all women. In 1995, "The Legacy Continues" was created, adding twenty-two women who were advocates for the cause who died of breast cancer during the first two years of the national exhibit tour.

First unveiled in 1993 in Washington, D.C., in the rotunda of the Russell Building of the United States Senate in May and later at the National Museum of Women in the Arts, the exhibit's national tour began in December of that year in Anchorage, Alaska. Installations in public spaces—museums, shopping malls, hospitals, and conference centers—have made it possible for tens of thousands of people to view it. The exhibit has motivated viewers to take charge of their own health care as well as to become breast cancer activists.

The exhibit has a powerful impact. The photographs show women at the peak of their lives, smiling, often with their families. The texts allow us to glimpse into their lives. These women were advocates who spoke out about their own battles against breast cancer. Each of them is one of the forty-six thousand women who die of breast cancer each year.

COMMUNITY OUTREACH

Providers often believe in a mission of community health but often hardly have the resources to address it within their own walls, much less their service area. Community health issues should not be borne by providers alone for one primary reason: they cannot afford—nor is it their responsibility—to fix problems such as socioeconomic and educational disparities, and transportation and housing concerns. But they can help by collaborating with others in community outreach efforts.

What does community outreach have to do with women's health? Women are looking for health care providers who care about the person, her family, and her community. The wise health care provider will find ways to promote all that they are doing for the community.

Partners for a Healthy Nashville (PHN) is a good example of provider and business collaboration.[2] PHN is a public-private partnership of health care, business, government, and community leaders working together to improve the health status of the Nashville community. It has three categories of partners: founding partners (ranging from the Nashville Junior League and Chamber of Commerce to the Tennessee Nurses Association and local hospitals and medical centers), funding partners (three foundations), and Health Pulse Partners (local and regional associations).

PHN's vision is to position Nashville as a community that is nationally recognized for providing a supportive environment to area employers and community organizations for the enhancement of the health and well-being of their employees. As stated in the mission, all objectives will be accomplished through partnerships by facilitating and coordinating resources and working collaboratively with local businesses, health care organizations, government, and citizen groups to improve the health status of the community.

The not-for-profit organization is funded through public and private sources including member contributions, local foundations, and matching grants from the metropolitan government. PHN is currently governed by a thirty-member board of directors and is an affiliate of the Nashville Area Chamber of Commerce.

Partners for a Healthy Nashville has a five-year commitment to improving the overall health and quality of life in its community by focusing efforts on five critical issues and accompanying goals:

1. *Maternal and infant health:* Increase immunization rates for two-year-old children from 84 to 90 percent and reduce pregnancies among girls aged fifteen to seventeen from sixty-four per thousand to fifty per thousand.

2. *Violence:* Reduce the rate of violent crime by 25 percent.

3. *Tobacco:* Reduce tobacco use by youth under the age of twenty from 42 to 25 percent and increase the number of smoke-free public places and workplaces, both indoors and outdoors, by 15 percent.

4. *Clinical and community prevention services:* Increase the proportion of people who engage in regular physical activity at least three to five times per week from 35 to 48 percent and increase the proportion of women over forty who receive a mammogram within the year from 60 to 72 percent.

5. *Alcohol and other drugs:* Reduce deaths caused by alcohol- and drug-related motor vehicle crashes by 20 percent and reduce

alcohol- and drug abuse–related hospital emergency room visits by at least 20 percent.

To date, Partners for a Healthy Nashville has had a great impact. It improved the health and lives of over four hundred families through home visits by a thirty-five-member health corps. After two years include: 99 percent of children in those families are free from abuse and neglect, and 95 percent have received immunizations. Most of the children born with low birth weight doubled their weight in six months and tripled it by their first birthday. Adults have greater parenting skills and knowledge, and five family health-risk factors have been reduced. The project has been funded for an additional three years and is now operated by United Neighborhood Health Services, Inc.

Another project organized over a hundred resources and fifty consultants for eighty Metro High School wellness teachers and improved the quality of annual in-services. PHN also partnered with a local research firm to provide a comprehensive health risk survey of 2,700 Nashvillians.

At the Healthy Nashville: Summit '98, the room was full to capacity with the movers and shakers of health care as well as the media and local politicians. The progress report enabled all the partners to stand up and be recognized as local heroes. What about providers who had chosen not to participate? From a competitive standpoint, they lost out in terms of goodwill and heightened awareness. At some point they may have to explain to consumers why they decided not to join with others on behalf of the community.

FAMILY-CENTERED CARE

Female consumers between the ages of thirty-five and fifty are the ones most sought after. They are also members of the "sandwich generation"—that is, those who care for both their children and their parents. Today, the aging population gets a great deal of attention. Health care providers are trying to address its needs through everything from Medicare risk to alternative living businesses. The teenage population, however, does not receive as much attention. For one thing, providers do not usually get many upstream referrals from this age group. For another, anyone who has raised a teenager realizes that their problems are not easy to deal with.

But a provider seeking ways to stand out by committing to relationship-centered care should consider working within the community to address adolescent health issues. If you do a good job at it, the mothers in the community will take notice. Youth development initiatives can embody the best of community outreach, but they demand that the provider community become actively engaged in enterprises that span a life cycle and that can influence the family, community, and society.

Sounds too broad? Think focusing on adolescent health may have some merit but not sure where to begin? Look at what your local community service agencies are doing and then decide what resources you might provide to bolster their agendas. For instance, most hospitals have a cadre of strategic planners and marketers committed to analyzing market share and competitive dynamics. What if you volunteered those very same resources to assist a local agency with its strategic planning process? What if you came in to develop a system for benchmarking adolescent health status and then tracking outcomes?

An example brings this to life. Nashville's Oasis Center is a private, not-for-profit, community-based agency providing comprehensive youth development services to teens and their families.[3] Originally conceived as a drop-in center to provide counseling and crisis intervention for clients of all ages, from its beginning the center has focused on prevention and treatment with programs such as crisis counseling and school-based education to prevent drug and alcohol abuse. The Rap House opened in 1969 in response to concerns about drug use in the community and the incarceration of juvenile-status offenders in adult jails. A health clinic was added the following year, and a crisis shelter, Oasis House, opened in 1976. In the early 1980s, Oasis Center refocused its efforts from serving individuals of all ages to providing comprehensive services to meet the needs of teenagers and their families. By concentrating on teenagers, the center could serve adolescents at the point at which they are most likely to get off track.

In 1988, Oasis Center developed a five-year plan with the following administrative and service-related long-range goals:

- Identifying and filling service gaps
- Identifying and serving minorities
- Advocating for children and family service needs at all levels
- Continuing to use sound agency management
- Diversifying the program's funding base
- Obtaining permanent facilities
- Refining financial and data management systems

Its focus in 1992 was largely on helping teens as individuals rather than on serving families or a geographically concentrated community. Since then the center has added more family-focused programs.

The Oasis Center has won scores of awards, including the Hospital Corporation of America (HCA) Award of Achievement for Volunteer Excellence (1994) and the HCA Award of Achievement for Management Productivity (1995).

Many Oasis partners from the provider community became involved almost grudgingly. But now most say they have learned a lot about how to build a pragmatic and relatively seamless continuum of care. They believe that the effectiveness of the continuum was derived from an internal commitment to communication so that no one—no teen, no family member, no off-site member of the care team—was left out of the loop of care and intervention. How often can that be said of the loop between the doctor's offices, the ambulatory care facility, and the hospital?

Because of their exposure to the Oasis Center staff and community, these providers have a real-life understanding of what relationship-centered care really means. One vice president of a hospital management company said, "I have never witnessed such a systematic approach to pursuing a mission and modifying activities in response to outcomes. The difference is that the outcomes being evaluated have to do with the quality of a youth's life and the value that the services bring to a family. It has been a privilege for me to observe this system in action. It has also helped me generate a new commitment for collaborative interactions within our organization. By our association with the Oasis Center, I came to understand that when our organization brings our resources of capital and strategic thinking to the table we will leave with something that is too often missing in our current homogenized system of health care: we will leave believing that we have worked together for a common purpose and that what we have done will make a difference." When asked if he would publicly promote and market his involvement and contributions, his answer was simply: "Of course."

HOLISTIC HEALTH

In 1993, David Eisenberg shocked the mainstream medical community by publishing a study on alternative and complementary therapies. Several of his findings have gotten the attention of both mainstream medical providers and business health care decision makers:

- In 1990, Americans made an estimated 425 million visits to providers of unconventional therapies. This number exceeds the number of visits to all U.S. primary care physicians (388 million).

- Expenditures associated with use of unconventional therapy in 1990 amounted to approximately $13.7 billion, three-quarters of which ($10.3 billion) was paid out of pocket.

- Roughly one in four Americans who see their medical doctors for a serious health problem are using a complementary therapy in addition to conventional medicine for that problem, and seven of ten who do so don't tell their doctor.

- The use of complementary therapies is not limited to the person's principal medical conditions. From an analysis profiling the respondents' utilization patterns, Eisenberg inferred that a substantial amount of complementary therapy is for nonserious medical conditions, health promotion, or disease prevention.[4]

Suddenly, the use of alternative or complementary therapies began to be regarded with more respect and interest. Some old-school physicians still remained wary and warned against voodoo cures, but some astute health care business decision makers looked at the shrinking revenues for their current lines of services and began to wonder if there might be an opportunity in the wings.

In 1998, John A. Astin of the Stanford Center for Research in Disease Prevention conducted a study to determine who uses alternative medicine and why. A total of 1,035 people were surveyed, and three theories to explain alternative medicine usage were tested:

- Patients are dissatisfied with conventional treatment.

- Patients see alternative treatments as offering more personal autonomy and control.

- Alternative therapies are more compatible with the patient's values.

Forty percent of respondents reported using some form of complementary medicine in the past year. Education was the number one sociodemographic variable that predicted complementary medicine usage.

Those with less than optimum health were also more likely to be users. The most frequently cited health problems treated with complementary medicine were chronic pain, anxiety, chronic fatigue syndrome, sprains and muscle strains, addictive problems, arthritis, and headaches.

The majority of complementary medicine users also find such therapies to be more congruent with their own values and beliefs. They tend to hold a philosophical orientation toward health that can be described as holistic. Dissatisfaction with conventional medicine did not predict alternative medicine usage.[5]

Women are particularly recognized for having a holistic orientation. OB/GYNs who survey their clients sometimes consider how to add a menu of holistic services to their practice, including massage, nutritional care, and aromatherapy. These physicians are motivated by two facts: their patients are willing to walk through another door to receive alternative services, and they are willing to pay cash for them.

But alternative therapy should not be regarded as the next gravy train for health care. Rina K. Spence discovered this when she opened the Spence Centers for Women's Health in Boston. She anticipated that alternative and complementary services would create a solid new revenue stream, but later sold her centers because they never truly realized the investors' expectations for return on investment. They can, however, be one way to broaden a base of primary care services and respond to consumer demand.

A widely recognized leader in the field of holistic health is Christiane Northrup, a board-certified OB/GYN and clinical assistant professor of obstetrics and gynecology at the University of Vermont College of Medicine's Maine Medical Center. She graduated from Dartmouth Medical School and completed her residency in OB/GYN at Tufts New England Medical Center Affiliated Hospitals, but her journey as a medical practitioner did not end with degrees, licenses, and a successful career. Sensing a deep need for change in the way medicine deals with people in general and women in particular, Northrup helped found Women to Women, an innovative health care center for women in Yarmouth, Maine that blends allopathic and alternative treatments. With the same goal in mind, she wrote *Women's Bodies, Women's Wisdom: Creating Emotional and Physical Health and Healing* (Bantam, 1994) and edits *Health Wisdom for Women*, a newsletter about women's health. A sample table of contents for one of these newsletters might include the following:

• Do you know what is really causing your symptoms? A multiple-choice quiz.

• Is your doctor listening to you?

• Five common recommendations that could be wrong for you!

• Do you love or hate your body?

• Five things you should know about diet and weight loss!

• How the female brain is different from men's.

• What doctors don't know about menopause.

• How to awaken your female intuition to help yourself.

• Positive emotions that can balance your hormones.

• How to program your mind for joy and healing.

If holistic health leaves you skeptical, you're not alone. But when you move beyond a holistic mind-body approach and add in a spiritual dimension, there is even more new data to consider.

Older patients with some religious link sliced hospital stays by more than half, according to a study conducted at Duke University Medical Center. Patients aged sixty or older with no religious affiliation spent an average of twenty-five days in the hospital, compared to eleven days for patients with some religious denomination, found Duke physicians Harold G. Koenig and David B. Larson, also president of the Washington, D.C.-based National Institute for Health care Research.

Additionally, researchers found that religious affiliation lowered the probability of being hospitalized. Patients who attend religious services once a week or more were 56 percent less likely to have been hospitalized the previous year than those who attend less frequently. After controlling for factors such as age, physical functioning, and severity of illness, researchers determined that patients who attend religious services weekly or more often are still 43 percent less likely to have been hospitalized in the past year, according to a study published in the October 1998 *Southern Medical Journal*.

The study examined the relationship between religious participation and affiliation and use of acute hospital services in 542 patients aged sixty or older admitted to Duke University Medical Center. Finding a factor such as religious commitment that drastically cuts frequency and length of hospital stays among elderly has potentially huge cost saving benefits.[6]

SUMMARY

According to Joan Borysenko, cofounder and former director of the Mind/Body Clinic at the New England Deaconess Hospital of Harvard Medical School, the quiet revolution in health care became public with the results of Eisenberg's Harvard study showing that a third of all Americans use some form of alternative medicine. In fact, more people sought an alternative practitioner than a primary care physician. Although these people may not have told their physicians what they were doing, they didn't abandon allopathic medicine. Providers are now challenged to explore integrative medicine—the use of both allopathic and alternative methods—and the difference between them. The former is based on a tremendously useful and important but sometimes limited view of the body as a machine. The latter is based on the fascinating and also sometimes limited notion that the body is a system of energy and that stimulation of that life-force energy is vital to healing. Those providers who excel in meeting the needs of their consumers will need to develop a comprehensive framework for integrative medicine that spans psychoneuroimmunology, psychocardiology, the mind-body connection, and the role of spirituality in the healing process.

Many hospitals and health systems are now embracing what is being called integrated medicine, a health care services approach that blends state-of-the-art conventional medicine with complementary or alternative approaches and an openness to acknowledging a spiritual dimension of care. The evidence is still being harnessed regarding the depth of replacement revenue that may be garnered or the true cost benefits of such an integrated approach, but patients are reporting that they appreciate the opportunity to participate in their own care and healing. Relationship-centered care means that the patient is involved and informed all along the way. He or she participates and decides rather than sits, waits, and passively receives. By opening your organization up to exploring some of these new paradigms, you may find that you create a venue that mitigates some of the depersonalization inherent in the current managed care environment and, in addition, you may reap some surprising benefits.

Notes

1. For more information on "The Face of Breast Cancer: A Photographic Essay," contact the National Breast Cancer Coalition Fund, 1707 L Street N.W., Suite 1060, Washington, DC 20036; phone: (202) 296–7477.

2. For more information on Partners for a Healthy Nashville, contact Joanne F. Pulles, Executive Director, 161 Fourth Ave. N., Nashville, TN 37219; phone: (615) 259–4728; e-mail: <jpulles@nashvillechamber.com>.

3. Burt, M. R., Resnick, G., and Novick, E. R.. "Building Supportive Communities for At-Risk Adolescents: It Takes More Than Services." *Advanced Practice Nursing Quarterly,*1998, *2*(4), 44–50.

4. Eisenberg, D. "Unconventional Medicine in the United States." *New England Journal of Medicine,* 1993, *328*(4), 246–251.

5. Astin, J. A. "Who Uses Complementary Medicine?" *Journal of the American Medical Association,* 1998, *279,* 1548–1553.

6. "Study Shows Religious Elderly Shrink Hospital Stays by 2 to 1." U.S. Newswire via NewsEdge Corp., Washington, D.C., Oct. 13, 1998.

CHAPTER NINETEEN

Conclusion

Genie James

———⁓⁓⁓———

Can hospitals and health systems win in the women's health care marketplace? Absolutely—if their strategy focuses on women's health and needs. That means embracing much more than reproductive medicine and gynecology; it means integrating women's health concerns across the continuum of care. How then should providers look at women's health as a long-term strategic initiative? The relationship between provider and patient must be expanded. The focus should not be solely on disease, but on health, well-being, and quality of life throughout a woman's lifetime.

The foundation for adult women's health is built in infancy and childhood, shaped by parents and buttressed by siblings, relatives, friends, and institutions such as churches, schools, and community organizations. Health care providers can and should help support and sustain all of these.

Unfortunately, according to Bill Bates, MD, "Many in modern American society lack the positive influence of parents, family members and friends. Health care providers can help fill in those blank spots by focusing on the fullness of life rather than on treatment of disease only. Health care institutions that can break from their traditional roles of treating disease and expand to promoting health will achieve greater financial success and will gain a competitive edge in the fragmented health care market. Physicians, HMOs, and hospitals cannot take on the responsibilities of family, church, school, and other organizations, but they can augment them. That is where health care providers can help people navigate the continuum of life."

If providers recognize and commit aggressively to this credo as being a long-term business opportunity, they will have customers for life. It is one motive for developing a new model for health services delivery that has a social conscience. Indeed, both economic and demographic factors demand a focus on women's health.

According to a report by Boston-based consultant firm Marketing to Women, women make at least 75 percent of consumer health care decisions, including those for their families. Beyond their clout in family decisions, however, women who are satisfied with their own health care can become a source of recurring revenue for providers. Their loyalty can pay dividends over decades.

Government, of course, remains a critical variable. Even in the increasingly aggressive managed care environment, women's health issues more often than not derive support from state and federal legislators. Federal dollars are finally being directed to women's health research. More important, lawmakers now recognize that passing legislation that can help keep mothers and wives alive and well will be highly visible and will help them to remain close to their voting public's hearts. They are thus quick to champion women's health issues.

Although they are a major economic force in health care, research shows that women have become increasingly dissatisfied with what has been traditionally available. Women have begun to demand medical solutions tailored especially for them, and providers are responding. What women want today is simple:

- Education and information about their health
- Convenient diagnostic and clinical services, and easy access to the care they need
- Sensitive treatment by health care providers

As the health care industry struggles to redefine itself in a new reimbursement environment, expensive technology is no longer the best way to hook new patients in a competitive marketplace. In fact, with managed care's strict approach to utilization management, providers are challenged to transition health care delivery from acute care services to models of care promoting prevention, wellness, and a sense of well-being. Consequently, industry leaders have a rabid desire to build a matrix that integrates supply-demand analysis with reimbursement projections. Everyone in the health care business is trying to figure out how to make money when the margins are so slim.

No other market segment is as potent as that of the female customer. It is a base of business that has yet to be fully realized. Women are taking the lead in defining what health care means to them and what it should deliver to their families. Meeting their needs and motivating them as customers is certainly a challenge, yet some industry leaders are learning to do so and profiting as they go.

From the beginning, this book emphasizes the critical importance of a customer-focused strategy. And it has discussed the following points:

- The average customer is female.
- She knows that she is a customer.
- She knows what she wants.
- She expects her managed care provider to pay for the care she wants.
- But if not, for services such as complementary medicine, nutritional therapy, cosmetic surgery, and weight loss programs, she is willing to pay out of her own pocket.

Also, this book proposes that any successful health care program must satisfy this equation:

$$\text{demographics} \times \text{dollars} \times \text{consumer demand} =$$
$$\text{product and services design} + \text{delivery and distribution}$$

Given that women are the majority now and that they expect providers to attend to their needs in new and better ways than ever before, it seems obvious that providers must attend to them. Women are no longer a market niche; providers who look only at reimbursement for reproductive services and gynecological surgeries will suffer in the long run.

If you, however—as a strategic thinker and responsible decision maker—understand how employer initiatives, Medicare strategies, movement toward new retail business lines, and your mission to address the needs of your community all come together, then you realize that women's health care is a seminal component of your long-term strategy for success.

This book offers practical models for moving past the organizational structures of IPAs, IDSs, and MCOs in order to return to a market-driven approach to capitalizing on consumer supply and demand. It looks at the revenue opportunity for both managed care risk taking and fee-for-service retail opportunities. Savvy health care decision makers are aware that a move toward consumer orientation means applying new skill sets as well as tried-and-true business principles. As Regina Herzlinger says, "The key to this entrepreneurial revolution is consumer control of the health care system."[1] Survival requires that the health care industry figure out how to respond to the consumer who demands information, convenience, and customized care while creating seamless systems offering the most advanced technology at the lowest cost. Acknowledging the import of a consumer-driven strategy logically leads decision makers back to the average consumer: the female in the market service area. With this logic, it should now be a given that a women's health strategy has the potential to move the health care industry from stagnation to innovation.

Note

1. Herzlinger, R. *Market Driven Health Care: Who Wins, Who Loses in the Transformation of America's Largest Service Industry.* Reading, Mass.: Perseus Books, 1997, p. xx.

~~~ Index